YOUR PREGNANCY . . .

What's it going to cost you? • Can you be stylish with a bump on your belly? • When do you switch from career girl to fulltime expectant mother? • How to beat the postpartum blues • What you should know about your obstetrician and your hospital • How—and when—to plan a perfect nursery • Natural childbirth for you? • All about maternity clothes • Your hospital suitcase • Do you tip the nurses? • How to photograph your newborn • Will you need a baby nurse? • The right name for your baby—when and how to choose it . . .

And more. Much more!

PREGNANCY NOTEBOOK

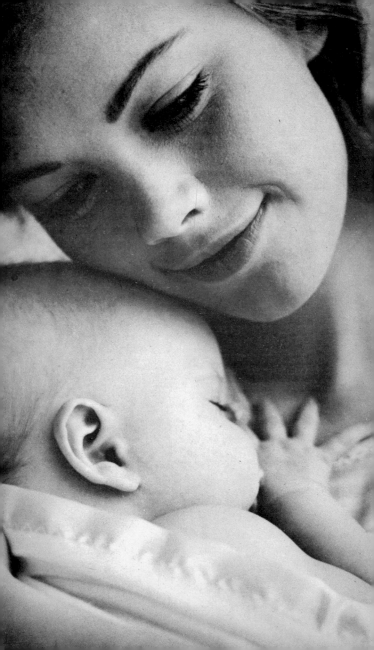

pregnancy notebook

by Marcia Colman Morton

BANTAM BOOKS · TORONTO · NEW YORK · LONDON

PREGNANCY NOTEBOOK
A Bantam Book

PRINTING HISTORY
Workman edition / July 1972

Bantam edition / October 1972

2nd printing .... December 1973	*4th printing .... April 1977*
3rd printing ..... November 1975	*5th printing .... August 1978*
6th printing ...... June 1980	

Published simultaneously in the United States and Canada

Bantam Books are published by Bantam Books, Inc. Its trade-
mark, consisting of the words ''Bantam Books'' and the por-
trayal of a bantam, is Registered in U.S. Patent and Trademark
Office and in other countries. Marca Registrada. Bantam
Books, Inc., 666 Fifth Avenue, New York, New York 10019.

PRINTED IN THE UNITED STATES OF AMERICA

15 14 13 12 11 10 9 8 7 6

This book is dedicated to
Dr. Jaffin, Dr. Moss and Mr. Morton
in gratitude for
a delightful pregnancy

acknowledgments

For their help to me in preparing this book I'd like to thank Mrs. Ruth W. Whitney of Glamour Magazine and Professor Lewis P. Lipsitt who provided me with data from his Child Study Center at Brown University.

And, especially, Mrs. Hermione Thomas, who generously shared with me all her experience and wisdom as the kind of maternity nurse every pregnant woman would be lucky to meet.

M.M.

contents

introduction

Getting ready to have a baby takes a lot of your time—think of all the daydreaming and wondering and imagining you have to do. But you also have to do a great many earthbound, reality things, for earthbound you and for that baby who's going to be very much a reality before you know it. He or she—let's call it "it" for now—will need so much. And *you* will need time for so many errands and chores if everything is to be ready and waiting for your baby, and comfortable for your husband, and pleasant for all other interested parties (like your older children, and plants, and pets, and friends, and family).

That's the reason for this book. You could make lists for yourself on the backs of old envelopes, tack up reminder notes all over the house . . . only to find yourself even more breathless in this already breathless time in your life. Instead, it's all here: a timetable of things to do at the most logical time to do them, with detailed discussions of each separate piece of planning, from arranging for a baby nurse to re-arranging your hair-do to balance the Bump, plus space for making your own lists and notes. With this book, you can gradually organize your new life over the months, not in a flurried last few days.

Obviously you're not a Boy Scout, but you can borrow their motto right now: Be Prepared. Early in your pregnancy, read this book through so you'll

know the jobs that are ahead of you. Then reread
appropriate sections as you tackle each separate
piece of planning.

Don't leave *anything* for the end sprint. Because
even in this scientific age, babies aborning have been
known to sometimes dilly-dally and sometimes jump
the gun. Of course your doctor uses all his science
and experience in giving you a probable birth date,
but just in case you've got a fast starter in there, get
everything ready for "it" early.

I know whereof I speak. When I was pregnant I
had a routine RH-negative problem, so the doctor
decided my baby should be born a couple of weeks
early when the proper treatment would be most
simple. He gave me a deadline—a Friday in the ninth
month—for giving nature a chance to cooperate.
Came that Friday, the doctor assured me that nature
was not cooperating. "Into the hospital Monday,"
he said. "We'll induce labor."

Which I thought was sort of nice, in a way. I
wouldn't have to sit around for several more weeks,
just me and the calendar and that packed, waiting
suitcase. I'd just prepare everything neatly over the
weekend. I made a confident little schedule for myself. Friday night: dinner and an evening with friends.
Saturday afternoon: stock the refrigerator and freezer
for my husband's lonesome week. Saturday evening:
manicure, pedicure, wash and set my hair. Sunday:
pack my suitcase while my favorite records played.
Sunday night: get to sleep early to be in fighting trim
for Monday.

Ha! By Monday I was the messy-haired, ragged-
nailed mother of a two-day-old daughter.

I got to bed late Friday after the long evening
with friends—only to be awakened a few hours later

by clear indications that nature, after all, was co-operating. I phoned the doctor, and though he was doubtful he did allow as how he might as well have a look. Why didn't I mosey on over to his office?

I woke my husband and invited him to join me, grabbed my natural-childbirth lemon candies (just in case), and the pocket make-up kit my beautiful actress friend had given me as *the* hospital necessity. And off I went to prove my point to the doctor.

"Well, you're right," he said. "Labor's going to start pretty soon. You'd better go to the hospital."

"But nobody goes to the hospital to have a baby without a suitcase," I said.

"You are," he said.

So there I lay, timing contractions, taking deep breaths and rubbing my belly as the natural-childbirth nurse had taught me, all the while dictating busy lists to my husband: "My make-up is on my dressing table. I'll need the face cream in the pink jar and the pale lipstick that says Bronze Natural on the bottom—it's in a tortoise-shell case. My new nightgowns are in my clothes cupboard, third—no, fourth shelf down. They're all in plastic bags, they're the ones you won't recognize. And my new house slippers, they're yellow and have no backs—not my old black ballet slippers. Oh, and I forgot my hairbrush—"

I also had to tell him about the casserole and layer cake my neighbor had left in our freezer for her dinner party that night. "—and maybe you'd better get yourself invited to help eat the casserole, there's nothing at home unless you wouldn't mind sardines."

You see what I mean. I should have packed my suitcase the day I entered the ninth month of my pregnancy. I should have stocked our larder. I should have— I should have had a book like this one. A book that organizes all the must-remember things into logical chapters and handy lists. A book that also, while we're at it, points out all the things you can do through your entire pregnancy to be a charming, efficient, pretty, unflurried and just altogether marvelous mother-to-be. But I never found such a book. So I wrote this one, for you.

part one

the first three months

chapter one
preliminary considerations

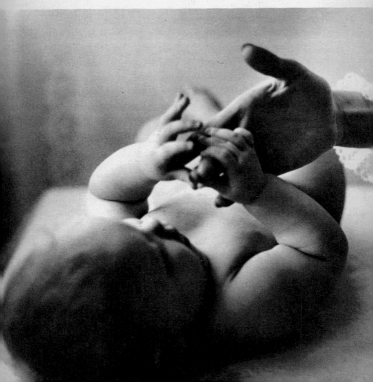

WHAT WILL IT COST YOU?

First things first, right? In fact, before you ever arrived at the interesting condition in which you now find yourself—pregnant I mean—ideally you should have considered the facts and figures this chapter deals with. That is, how much is this little venture going to cost you and Daddy?

According to figures from recent surveys,* the answer is $1,735—at least. It breaks down like this:

---

* Figures compiled from projections and surveys conducted by the Health Insurance Institute, the American Hospital Association, The American College of Obstetrics and Gynecology, and *Medical Economics*. The figures are valid as of early 1972, but, like all costs in our inflationary economy, they are likely to go up.

1. HOSPITAL CARE   **$715**
    5 days at $93.00 per day for a semi-private
       room (2 in a room)   **$465**
    Delivery room charge   100
    Nursery for 5 days at $27.00 per day   135
    Circumcision set-up   15

2. MEDICAL CARE   **$335**
    Obstetrician   275
    Circumcision fee   35
    Pediatrician's newborn care   25

3. INFANT'S LAYETTE   **$520**
    Basic wardrobe   70
    Nursery items   340
    Utensils, bath items, miscellaneous   110

4. MATERNITY CLOTHING   **$165**

                                                      $1,735

And these figures are, believe it or not, conservative.
If you live in a large city in a state like New York or
California, your hospital and doctor bills will be
higher simply because large cities are more expensive generally. Should you need a Caesarean delivery you'll be in the hospital for about eight days
which will cost you more. If you choose to splurge
on a private room or need to stay somewhat longer
than the standard four or five days, or if you or
your baby requires special hospital services—up,
up, up go the prices.

    As for figures 3 and 4, they really are minimal.
You'd be more realistic to budget a thousand dollars for those items, unless you can count on hand-

me-downs for maternity party clothes and for such things as a playpen, door guards, a travel carriage—items that make baby's life and yours more comfortable in his early months. What's more, nowhere in the surveys is there an estimate for extra domestic help, or diapers which are a one-year running expense that can go as high as two hundred and fifty dollars (the figures take you through the first week only), or the cost of moving to larger quarters. . . .

But wait, there's help. Your health-insurance plan may pay for a good part of items 1 and 2. Check now to see how much your present policy covers. If the answer is—sigh!—nothing, it's probably too late to change things for this pregnancy. Many insurance companies insist that maternity coverage be arranged before conception. At the very least, though, this is a good time to get your health insurance in order for your next pregnancy.

If you have neither insurance coverage nor cash on hand to take care of that $1,735, start planning now how to budget for some of it, borrow the rest of it, and otherwise prepare for the little stack of bills the stork will deposit right along with baby.

If you can't manage the fees for a private obstetrician and hospital, remember that clinic care at a good hospital, especially one affiliated with a medical school, is as good as the care of a private obstetrician. In every city there are clinics run by voluntary hospitals, subsidized by the city, community, or church, that offer less costly care. The essential difference is that you do not have a choice of doctors, but instead are taken care of by the house staff under the supervision of an attending doctor. For instance, like most fine doctors, my own excellent, high-priced, private obstetricians devote several mornings a week to hospital work and are on call at all times for consultation. And even if your bed is in a ward rather than a semi-private room, you'll still have the benefit of the same delivery room, the same expert techniques, the same accumulated knowledge of the hospital's staff of childbirth specialists ready to take care of you and your newborn baby.

So, though money and budget are something to think about, they don't have to be a hang-up. Just plan now on the best way for you to obtain everything you and baby will need. When you know what hospital you'll be going to, ask the admitting office for an estimate of your hospital costs. Ask them for all alternative choices in costs as well as all charges for extra services as your doctor foresees them. Of course, at this point, they can only give you an estimate, but at least you'll have the most knowledgeable estimate possible to guide you in your planning. Enter these estimates on the list of expenses, page 85. When you know what kind of room you'll want let your doctor know so he can reserve a hospital bed for you.

CHOOSING YOUR OBSTETRICIAN AND HOSPITAL

If you don't already have a regular gynecologist/obstetrician, finding one is your first pregnancy job. You want the best qualified, most experienced doctor there is. Probably your general practitioner or family internist will refer you to his most trusted obstetrical colleague. Or your mother or older sister or friend-who-had-a-baby-last-year will urge you to get *her* wonderful doctor to oversee your pregnancy and delivery. You can also call your local county medical society, or go right to the best hospital in your community and ask for a list of the doctors on the obstetrics staff.

Whichever guide you follow, the important thing is to be sure your obstetrician's medical credentials are unimpeachable. His postgraduate training as a specialist should have been at a first-class hospital and he should be on the staff of one of the top hospitals in town. Check him out with a doctor you already know and trust or with your local medical society. Then, on your very first visit, decide if you feel comfortable with him; if you find him kind and sympathetic and compatible—because you and he will be collaborators on a months-long project.

I, for instance, did not feel at ease with the first obstetrician to whom I was referred. He was an excellent doctor but some of the attitudes he expressed seemed old-fashioned to me. I didn't feel I would be able to talk freely with him through all my visits. So I asked *everyone* about obstetricians. When four separate women all recommended the same pair of doctors (gynecologists often work as a duet so that one of them is always sure to be available when your baby decides to be born), I felt that was pretty impressive. First I got my internist's medical approval; then I made an appointment, found them very congenial and never regretted my switch.

Among the factors that will tell you whether the doctor is right for you: if you are thinking of using natural childbirth, make sure on your first visit that your doctor will cooperate. Find out if one of *his* basic attitudes conflicts with one of *yours*—does he disapprove, say, of bottle-feeding or rooming-in or any other maternal notion you've set your heart on? Is he easy to talk to? Does he practice reasonably

near your home so that you can get to his office
easily? Is he always reachable by telephone?

Ask him for a clear statement of the obstetrician's
total fee for pre- and post-natal care plus delivery.
Also find out what hospital he uses, or later you may
be disappointed to discover, too late, that his hospital does not match your dream of motherhood. Consider, for instance, whether you may want rooming-in
for your baby (page 107) or a Father Hour (page
108). Not all hospitals offer these facilities. If they're
very important to you, try to find a hospital that has
them. If your pregnancy poses any special problems,
check to see that the hospital is equipped to deal
with them. Find out which hospital reasonably near
you (it shouldn't be more than a half-hour drive
away) provides the services you want, and try to
match up obstetrician and hospital for the best possible combination.

If you will be using a clinic instead of a private
obstetrician, choose the clinic—and the hospital it
is a part of—by the same criteria. Ask your present
doctor, your relatives and your friends for their
experiences. And if you're not happy with your
first choice, remember that you can always go elsewhere.

Enter the name, address and phone number of the
clinic or your obstetrician, and those of the hospital,
in the space provided for them in the middle of the
book. Also write down your appointments on the
Pregnancy Calendar on page 66. During the first
five months, appointments are usually monthly, during the next two months, semi-monthly, and during
the final three months, weekly. Jot down in the appropriate space any questions you want to ask your
doctor on your next visit. Circle your due date, it's
a singular day.

NATURAL CHILDBIRTH

If you're afraid, don't be ashamed to admit it to yourself or anyone else. Almost every expectant mother worries. Studies have shown that pregnant women even dream about their fears. And yet their fears have less basis in fact than they *ever* dreamed.

The trouble stems from the way girls used to be brought up. Until your generation, women were conditioned for childbirth only with scare stories, never with truthful reassurance. Dire hints mothers passed along to daughters, novels featuring what was always called "the agony of birth," old cornball movies where the off-screen mother filled the sound track with screams and the doctor helped her with "plenty of hot water!" and very little else . . . No wonder women went into labor with every nerve jangling, every muscle clenched, creating pain even where there was none.

Today we're beginning to understand how unfrightening and comfortable childbirth can be. Not only are medications highly developed for easing you through when necessary, but the medications themselves are often rendered unnecessary by something much better. In a speech before the World Congress of Gynecology and Obstetrics in 1970, the eminent anesthesiologist, Dr. Bradley E. Smith, explained why his own profession—the administering of anesthesia—was becoming less and less necessary for childbirth. Much of the pain during labor and delivery, he noted, *is a result of fear*. Anything a doctor can give his patient "psychoprophylactically"—that means, in plain language, to calm her down mentally —"including a pat on the head and verbal assurance, will help reduce the amount of sedation she needs."

That's why you're so lucky to be pregnant now. It's only since 1950 that obstetricians have developed the techniques commonly known as natural child-birth or educated childbirth—an uncomplicated use of proper breathing, relaxation and exercise to condition your childbirth muscles and reflexes to do their work efficiently. If "a pat on the head and verbal assurance" can reduce pain for most women, think what this specialized training can accomplish!

As a young woman of the 1970's, you've probably already been given some informal anti-fear training along with the scare stories of olden days. You've heard from friends about childbirth being—surprise, thank God!, surprise—more a thrilling joy than anything else. Take it from me, a card-carrying coward, it's true. Most ladies who advise trying natural childbirth sound like real strong sisters—at least they always did to me, and I always dismissed their words with the certainty that *I* could never go through with that spartan idiocy. But as soon as I was pregnant, I decided to take the training anyway, just because, as a coward, I wanted to do everything I could to make the pain less—*please!*

It worked. The pain was less—it was non-existent for me. In spite of my pre-training fears, plus the fact that I was over 35 and having my first baby, I was able to stay alert and undrugged through an incredibly comfortable labor and have mild medication only at the end for delivery.

A nurse friend of mine, when she learned that I was writing this book, implored me to make the point that you needn't go into natural-childbirth training with the rigid resolve to follow it through all the way to delivery. Tragically, that misconception stops a lot of girls. Just proceed on the assumption that the techniques will help you as far as you care to go, and then you can use medication as so many natural-childbirth trainees do. Or you may amaze yourself by wanting to stay awake for the entire birth, as many other women do nowadays. (I felt that I could have, except that we knew beforehand that my baby would have to be delivered fast for the RH treatment it would need immediately.)

Whatever you do, do *not* refuse even to investigate this wonderful new technique invented for women at last. Do some reading to become familiar with the subject. *Thank you, Dr. Lamaze* by Marjorie Karmel is a charmingly written personal memoir and practical guide dedicated to the French obstetrician who introduced the author—and indeed the entire Western world—to the idea of painless childbirth. *Six Practical Lessons for an Easier Childbirth* by Elisabeth Bing is exactly what its title says—a book version, with many helpful photographs, of the course given by the author who is one of America's leading teachers of the Lamaze method. Both books are widely available in paperback for about a dollar. (For more on natural childbirth see page 102.)

SEE YOUR DENTIST

After your obstetrician says, "Yes, you're pregnant," his next words will probably be, "See your dentist!" The growing fetus dips lustily into your calcium reserve, and your own teeth may suffer. But not if you're a good girl and make a pregnancy-long schedule of appointments with your dentist. Enter them on the Pregnancy Calendar and add your dentist's name, address and phone number to your address list on page 82.

INCOME-TAX DEDUCTIONS

Save receipts for everything you spend on your pregnancy. With the exception of baby and maternity clothes and nursery furniture, they're almost all deductible. If you require any special expenditures, get a note from your doctor explaining that these are necessary to your health and baby's health and attach it to your income-tax form.

Deductions include all doctor or clinic, dentist, and hospital fees you pay for yourself and your baby, all drug bills, and the cost of any tests or X-rays for which you aren't covered. Also included are the wages for any nurse who takes care of you before or after your baby is born, and all traveling expenses to doctor and hospital, whether by ambulance, taxi, bus or private car. One-half of your insurance premiums can be deducted, and state and city sales tax (you're bound to have a number of large purchases), and the interest paid on any loan you've had to take out and on anything bought on time. Under the latest Tax Reform Act, passed in December 1971, you can now deduct for the cost of household help if you have a child at home and, when the time comes, the cost of a childcare center. The amount you are able to deduct depends on your income, so check with your accountant or your local Internal Revenue Service. Of course, you are also entitled to a personal exemption for your new dependent. Under this same Tax Reform Act the rate of the exemption has gone up. If your baby is born before midnight of December 31, 1972, you are entitled to a $750 exemption (as a married couple with one child your total tax exemption would be $2250—$750 × 3). As of this writing, it has yet to be determined if the figure will stay the same or go up in 1973 and 1974. So, again, check with the Internal Revenue Service.

Record your expenses in the space provided for them on page 86.

THE NEWBORN NURSE

One thing you and baby don't *need,* but is mighty nice to have, is that supreme luxury known as a newborn nurse. She's the lady, generally mature, who has had special training in the care of newborns. And, oh, her experience! She's prone to statements beginning, "Well, with my 156 *other* babies, I always did it this way. . . ."

But she's wonderful. She knows just how to bathe a five-day-old, just how to dress him for every temperature change, just exactly how hungry he is how often, just what every cry means, how to treat every little rash . . . she knows everything! She's a treasure, and she's expensive. The going rate in New York City is about $145 for a six-day week, proportionately lower in less expensive parts of the country.

If you can afford a newborn nurse, you can hire her either through an employment agency specializing in these ladies or through personal recommendation. Most women prefer the second method. For the floundering mother-to-be, nothing is more reassuring than the fervent reference given by a good nurse's grateful graduate: "Nanny taught me everything I know! A rock!"

Start asking your friends as soon as you're pregnant, and interview every nurse you hear well of. Check references thoroughly and realistically, but also look the candidates over carefully. Draw them out in conversation. The nurse's personality is very important. She will be living with you and sharing with you one of the most intense, intimate experiences of your life—the care of your tiny new child. She will be—for the days or weeks or months she lives in your home—your teacher, mother, sister, friend, or enemy when you disagree over what to do for baby.

When you do find the nurse whose references are irreproachable and whose personality seems compatible to yours, hire her immediately. (While you're deciding, keep notes on the candidates in the space provided for them on page 84). You should engage the booked-far-ahead personal-referral kind of nurse when you're about three months pregnant. If you wait longer, a more foresighted mother may already have booked the nurse you want for your delivery date. And you can always change your mind later— these ladies won't penalize you. They're so much in demand they can easily find replacement jobs.

If you don't want to make a choice so soon, whether for superstitious or practical reasons, whenever you feel ready ask your obstetrician and your friends about reputable nurses' employment agencies. The agencies almost always have several candidates available for you to interview. You can even call an agency from your hospital bed after the baby is born, and they'll generally have someone capable at your home within a couple of days.

If you do engage a nurse in advance, get her phone number immediately, both her home phone and her current job (naturally, the nurse's job phone number changes quite often). Give her your number as well, and ask her to phone you every month or so to give you her current job phone in case you need to get in touch with her. Tell her the date you expect her to start work, and the length of time you will want to employ her—anywhere from a few days to several months, depending on your finances and your family situation. Call her as soon as you have any change in expected birth date so that she can adjust her plans. And, of course, call her from the hospital to tell her the baby is here, what its sex is, and when she is to report for action. Most nurses enjoy coming to the hospital to escort you and baby home—a welcome help at that bustling hour.

Whatever you think now, you really will appreciate some help in your first maternal days. If you can't afford a newborn nurse, or if you would rather not have one—many mothers prefer to take total charge of the baby themselves—there are a number of excellent alternatives which you can arrange in the weeks just before your baby arrives: a week's visit from an experienced mother, aunt, or young grandmother, or daily drop-in visits if such relatives live nearby. A cleaning woman or a housekeeper hired full-time or part-time for those tiring first weeks would probably be even better. And most helpful of all is a hospital course in baby care for you and Daddy (see page 104).

chapter two

the pregnant you

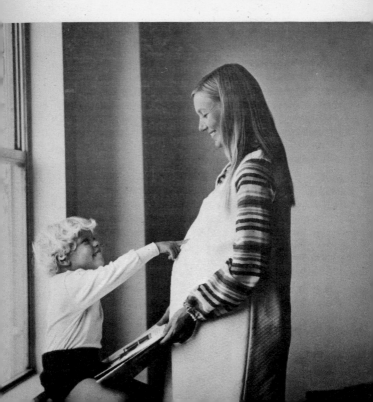

WORK

Unless your job is incredibly taxing, physically or mentally—or your pregnancy is that rare one requiring complete rest—if you're working when you get pregnant, the universal medical advice is to go right on working.

You and your doctor will agree on the right time for you to quit your job. This might be about the sixth month, to give you time to prepare your nursery and layette. Or you might be one of those ladies who, one bright morning, phones the office to explain she won't be in that day, having become a mother during the night.

One girl I worked with, a magazine editor, gave

birth the dawn before her magazine issue was going to press. Five hours later she was on the phone to her assistant with detailed instructions on how to complete the issue. She was back at her desk in time for the next issue.

Then there is the teacher in my daughter's nursery school. She quit at the end of the school year, five months pregnant and very pleased with her neat timing. But came September, her replacement was suddenly called out of the city, and though she was now eight months pregnant, the school board begged her to fill in, Bump and all, until a new replacement could be found. So there she was, practically till delivery day, teaching the four-year-olds Mother Goose, finger painting and where-babies-come-from. The kiddies loved it ("Just like Mommy!" they'd squeal) and so did their teacher.

There are many advantages to working your way through pregnancy. The money, of course; unless your husband is doing spectacularly well, you will certainly be able to use your salary toward all the new expenses.

Just as important is the morale boost a job can be. A job gives you *something else* interesting to think about, a reason to get up and get pretty each day, a proud feeling that you're cooking on all burners while fulfilling your most fundamental womanly drive. You'll be more relaxed about expecting a baby if it's not the only factor in your daily existence for nine whole months; if you don't merely lounge around the house daydreaming about coming events; if you lead as rich and varied a life as ever, with socializing and hobbies *and* a job. And, unlike my magazine-editor friend who was back at her desk at the first possible post-natal moment, you may very well call a halt in your working life during your children's early years. All the more reason, then, to enjoy your last months—for a while—as a career girl.

Not that you won't need to make some adjustments. Since you should have a daily walk, plan time for this on your lunch hour. If you're watching your weight and find you can't get low-calorie lunches at your usual luncheonette or restaurant, bring the cottage cheese and carrots from home to eat at your desk before or after your walk. If you suffer from morning sickness in your early pregnancy, try to arrange to get to the office after it's over. Or inform your employer of your problem so that it's understood you will adjourn to the ladies' room when necessary. Or discuss medication with your doctor. And if you and your doctor feel you should have an afternoon nap or rest, try to arrange with your employer how best to schedule this.

The very nature of your job may demand small changes in your work routine. In my late pregnancy I found it too hard on my back to type for the long periods I was accustomed to. So I simply worked at my typewriter for as long as it was comfortable, then did stand-up chores for a while to ease my back (rereading, penciling corrections), then sat down and typed some more. Think of ways to adjust your job duties.

Obviously, from all the foregoing, you'd better not try to keep your little secret from your boss. It'll be easier all around if you make your announcement as soon as possible. For you: freedom to plan small adjustments in your working day to accommodate your new physical state. For the boss: time to hire your replacement early enough so you can train her if necessary.

In some companies there are rules against the employment of pregnant women. In that case, find out quickly when you will have to leave. Which brings up the question of when you quit, and if and when you return to work. Start thinking early about both answers, in consultation with your doctor (for medical advice) and your husband (for budget and lifestyle considerations).

Whatever you decide, investigate your company's insurance coverage. Are you entitled to maternity benefits? Are these different for mothers who quit their jobs permanently and those who return to the company?

And don't forget one lovely fringe benefit of being a working mother-to-be. When the time comes for you to quit, your co-workers will almost certainly give you a baby shower, which should fill out some of your layette and nursery needs nicely.

PLAY

As with work, so with play. The tried-and-true obstetrical advice in modern times is to continue as physically active when you're pregnant as when you're not—subject, of course, to your doctor's opinion and to special facts in *your* pregnancy.

Do not follow a word of the following guide without first checking with your doctor on how it all applies to your very personal case. But on the whole, here's a sketch of what you can expect of your sports activity in a normal pregnancy.

If you are a tennis player, go on playing tennis, though in a somewhat milder form—that is, you won't run and leap for a really difficult ball. You don't want to get too tired.

Swimming is perfectly marvelous for you, at whatever level of competence you are generally used to. Walking is wonderful too, the only difficulty being with uphill climbs in the later months. Go as far and as high as you can without getting uncomfortably breathless.

Golf—great, though your swing may be thrown off a little by The Bump's extra weight and new center of gravity. If you're a dancer, go on with the dance. Ballerinas have often pirouetted into the seventh or eighth month. When I was pregnant, I was working on research about charity balls, and I danced, notebook in hand, through three separate evenings the week before my baby was born. There *was* a little problem in pointing The Bump sideward when I fox-trotted or waltzed with my husband. And I don't know that I'd be thrilled to see a very pregnant lady and Bump gyrating in frug-like rhythms. But dancing, like any moderate exercise, is healthy and morale-building.

If you haven't been involved in any sport, maybe now's the time to start. If you're an unathletic type with no specific preference, look into natural childbirth classes where you can get the exercise you need.

TRAVEL

Of course you can go anywhere you like for vacation or business, but you may prefer to stay rather close by your obstetrician. Small emergencies can arise where a comforting examination and reassurance from the doctor who knows your case can make all the psychological difference.

If you do plan to travel far, ask your doctor for the name, address and phone number(s) of a respected obstetrician at your destination. Give your doctor a few days' notice so he has time to inquire a bit for the right stand-in. Enter the new doctor's name, address and phone number on page 82. If you must undertake a journey after the seventh month, go the quickest and easiest way possible. Don't forget to take along your pregnancy paraphernalia— vitamins, medication, support stockings. . . .

DIET

Your eating habits in pregnancy have two aims: to nourish baby and you, and to keep you from gaining too much weight. Overweight is as unhealthy for you now as it is for anyone at any time. By the end of the nine months, your doctor will be pleased to see you gain no more than eighteen or twenty pounds.

But good nutrition is, if anything, even more important. Malnutrition in pregnancy leads directly, tragically, to a baby with a low IQ and poor physical development. High on your doctor's list of concerns will be your diet, and if you follow his advice you'll be fine on all counts. Keep notes on the foods he recommends you eat for nutrition and for cutting calories and get yourself a purse-size calorie-count booklet—they're available at most paperback stores.

A note on those legendary pre-natal food cravings you may find yourself subject to: According to recent studies, they are due to changes in the pregnant woman's sense of taste and smell.

POSTURE, HAIR AND SKIN CARE

Pregnant women, they say, look beautiful. Yes, well, it's true that from your fourth month on your complexion may have a radiance it never knew before, and *my* problem hair did go suddenly, unprecedentedly glossy and smooth without my usual cream treatments and so forth. A friend of mine says that, thank heavens, her leg hair is less abundant when she's pregnant—thank heavens because it's so much harder in the later months to lean over to shave. Another woman, who had her first baby at thirty, remembers that during her pregnancy, her tiny wrinkles disappeared and her skin took on a teenage glow.

But let's face it—we've all admired certain pregnant women for looking great, and been depressed by others who mope around looking dragged, uncared-for, plodding. Which way will *you* look? It's entirely up to you. If you give some thought and a little time to your beauty routines, you will be a joy to behold for your friends, for your husband, and for yourself.

The first thing, as every lovely woman knows, is inner attitude. You're happy, aren't you, about your exciting condition? That will show. It will show just as much as The Bump. Accept the fact that The Bump is with you, bigger every day for months. For these few months your style is not the golden girl in body shirt and hip-huggers. But it will be again, and in the meantime, you're attractive, you honest-and-truly are. Almost every man alive really does think that a pregnant woman is an esthetically delightful creature—even confirmed bachelors do. As for most women, the unpregnant look at the pregnant with either fond nostalgia or a hopeful eye to the future. Pregnant, you are beautiful, because you're a living example of the most thrilling human act.

And so your aim is not to ignore The Bump or pretend it's not there. Instead you want to stand proudly, walk gracefully, and groom the non-Bump areas lovingly.

Posture. This is your basic pregnant-beauty consideration. Exercises taught in natural childbirth classes are a tremendous help here. They improve your pre- *and* post-natal muscle tone. You will stand better, move better, feel better, *look* better, especially in the later months. Ask your doctor about this, and have him recommend a private or hospital class. Or perhaps he or his nurse can teach you exercises to do at home if you don't want to splurge on a course fee. In any case, he will advise you on how often, how much, and how late in your pregnancy you can exercise.

Hair. First of all, let's get the texture into condition. The hormone changes occurring in pregnancy can make dry or normal hair temporarily oily, and hair that is usually oily can become a real problem. In pregnancy, hair also tends to grow faster, and straighter, beginning in the fifth month.

In my case, all this was a great morale booster— my previously dry, too curly, slow-growing hair became a long, shining mane that was the glory of my pregnancy. In your case, you may not need or want the extra locks and over-straightness; so it's more frequent cutting and shaping for you! If you need to combat a sudden over-oiliness in your hair, use a special anti-oil shampoo, and shampoo more frequently. Use conditioners made for oily hair. Dry-shampooing for quick fix-ups are a help, as are between-shampoo settings with electric curlers which tend to dry out hair—a *good* thing for you right now. Bleach-streaking will also dry out an oily condition and is especially attractive on blondes.

Should your shiny hair turn suddenly dry and life-less, try brushing more often; use special shampoos made for dry hair; try cream rinses, oil treatments for your scalp, pomade-like hair dressings, and those special hair sprays that add highlights and sheen.

Don't choose this time to change your hair color completely with long-lasting dyes. If you don't like the results, you'll be depressed and have to go in for wearisome, expensive sessions with the hair-dresser to undo your mistake. Even if you love your new color, you may not have time to keep it up during your first busy weeks as a mother. You could find yourself walking around with that horror of horrors: a dye job growing out at the roots. How-ever, slightly brightened hair color is a good idea for the pregnant woman. You might try a shampoo-in color rinse for a glowing highlight.

Hair-do? Your object is to balance The Bump. The larger *it* gets, the tinier your head will look in comparison. Instinctively, pregnant women seem to switch to fuller, fluffier coiffures in the later months to achieve an esthetic balance. Experiment—with the aid of your hairdresser if possible—to achieve the most flattering coiffure. A practical consideration is to find a hair-do that does not require constant setting and attention. Hair-fussing will have a very low priority on your busy schedule those first weeks with baby. Look into those wonderful shaped cuts that need almost no setting, a particular boon during your hospital stay so you can look glamorous for visitors with only the aid of a comb and brush. Watch magazines and women's pages for hair-do's that seem right for you.

By the way, don't be surprised, after your baby is born, if your hair falls out in rather startling quantities. It's a common condition, and goes away a few months after childbirth when you'll get a nice new growth. Until then, either cut your hair short or wear it glossily pulled back with decorative bows and clips. To encourage hair stength during these months, stay away from harsh treatments like dyes and straighteners. Stick to hairbrush, mild shampoos and conditioners.

Skin care. Many pregnant women's complexions improve with pregnancy, taking on that vibrant glow, clearing up old problems of blackheads and pimples. But sometimes a mother-to-be with a previously trouble-free complexion suddenly develops an oil problem and starts breaking out like an adolescent with acne.

If this happens to you, discuss it with your obstetrician. He will either suggest new oil-cutting cleansers and medications for you, or he will refer you to a dermatologist who will diagnose the problem and prescribe treatment for it before it can do permanent damage. If, on the other hand, the hormone changes of pregnancy make your skin go dry, you should use soapless cleansers and moisturizing face creams. However, avoid using those with hormones in them. Itchy skin is also a common pregnant woman problem. Your doctor can usually prescribe medication to relieve it.

A lot of pregnancy chit-chat has to do with—
shudder!—stretch marks and the prevention thereof.
Girls tell each other about this or that magic po-
tion, and slather The Bump and adjoining areas
religiously each night and pray for the best. When I
brought up the subject with my own doctor, he said:
a) What's so bad about stretch marks, even in a
bikini? and b) It's up to nature—either you're prone
to stretch marks or you're not; slathering won't
change things.

I got annoyed at his lack of sympathy, and finally
got him to allow as how cocoa butter—very cheap,
and available at every drugstore—was as good as
anything more elaborate. I went ahead and slathered
enthusiastically, and I didn't get stretch marks. To
which he smiled indulgently and didn't say another
word. So, conscientiously, I'll put together medical
opinion and my own experience and advise: Right
on with the cocoa butter. At least you'll smell like a
chocolate bar.

Make-up. You will want your face to look brighter
to balance the eye-catching Bump and to counter a
tendency to look pale, tired, perhaps a little swollen.
Try more color in your eye shadow, soft color—pale
blue or green for light eyes, mauve or taupe for dark.
If you've never used eye shadow—at least not in the
daytime—now is the time to start. And definitely
use mascara with it, maybe even delicate false lashes
to draw attention to your eyes. Shape your brows
and have them colored—nothing does more to combat a wan look. Stroke on face blusher, maybe in a
tawnier shade than usual. And use lipstick even if
you've never done *that* before—the spot of color
will glow-up your whole face.

A flawlessly groomed pretty face makes all the difference in the world. You'll look great and you'll feel great . . . subtle, chic, glowing.

If you're not an old hand at the make-up table, ask an expert friend. Or get one of those free lessons offered in the cosmetics departments of large stores or beauty establishments. They throw in the advice session free if you buy a minimum amount of cosmetics—a very worthwhile investment. And in the beauty magazines you'll find at your hairdresser's, and the more thoughtful obstetricians' offices, you can always find articles on make-up often accompanied by demonstration photos.

Now just lean back and accept graciously the compliments about the marvelous new natural beauty you've achieved through pregnancy. And don't forget what you've learned—be a beautiful young mother too.

MATERNITY CLOTHES

One piece of advice I got—and you will get—from every woman who's ever been pregnant is: Don't buy a lot of maternity clothes. "A lot," of course, is relative to your social and economic circumstances. But what it means is buy the minimum, really, of what you need. I ignored this advice and splurged rather heavily within my income. I can now, from my own experience, join the chorus: Don't buy a lot of maternity clothes. If, like me, you disregard this universal wisdom, reread this paragraph after you've had your baby and see if you don't agree, after the fact, after all.

No matter what you tell yourself about wearing your maternity clothes Afterward, you won't—not with any degree of pleasure. No matter how fashionably cut they are, no matter how striking in color or fabric, no matter how supposedly convertible to the non-pregnant figure—you will be glad to see the last of them after your baby is born. If only in your mind, they will always retain the contour of The Bump.

Take me. I was pregnant in the year of the Tent. Remember the tent? A style everybody said was ideal for pregnant women? It was, and so I outfitted myself with four non-maternity evening tents for partygoing. They were very pretty and quite expensive, and I told everyone blithely how I would wear them for years. My previously pregnant friends smiled patiently.

By the time I had my baby, the tent had gone so far out of fashion you could find it only in thrift shops. In came evening pajamas and fitted pants suits. To get at least a little of my money's worth out of my extravagant tents, about the only thing I could do was to shorten them, buy belts for them, and wear them as tunics over slacks—feeling forever pregnant all the while. But I was too embarrassed to buy any of the mouth-watering new fashions until I'd worn my "wearable for years" maternity clothes at least a few times more. Thank heavens, soon afterward a tightly budgeted young bride I knew announced that she was expecting a baby. She couldn't get over my kindness in begging her to take —please!—my entire maternity wardrobe.

So the thing for you to do as soon as you've passed your third month is to look for friends like me— recently pregnant ladies who are fantastically eager to pass along (or at least lend until their next pregnancies) their maternity purchases, just to see them get enough use to justify their cost. Among certain close-knit groups, friends run a veritable lending-library of maternity clothes. Ascertain all your sources, and take everything the minute anyone offers it.

Go through your pre-pregnant wardrobe to see what you already own that's styled loose and easy enough to see you through mid-pregnancy—say, the start of the seventh month. Switch to these as soon as you begin to look like a sausage in your more fitted clothes, and try not to buy true maternity outfits until later as they are quickly outgrown. Put the fitted things away for post-pregnancy wear instead of stretching them irretrievably beyond Afterward use.

You may even find that some of your clothes will be wearable through your entire pregnancy. I happened to have three wool capes that saw me splendidly through mine. A full non-fitted coat or a wrap-around would do nicely. Check to see if you have any jumpers, dresses, dashikis and kaftans that could accommodate The Bump. Also overblouses, cut straight, full or A-line, anything Empire-style, ponchos and tunics.

The general rule about maternity clothes is: Don't rush into them, but don't wait too long. That is, start wearing them the minute you don't look attractive in anything else. But if you buy them too soon, you may be wasting your money. It all depends on the way *you* Bump. Some ladies stay small enough not to need special clothing ever. Others belong in real maternity garments from the fifth month on. Others outgrow them in a month. So unless you are rich enough to buy a new maternity wardrobe for every month of your pregnancy, I'd say shop for a dress or

whatever *as you need it*. Try to make it a test for
yourself to see if you can get by without shopping
until your sixth month. Of course, if you've been un-
lucky in your search for hand-me-downs, or if your
closet has been singularly unresourceful, of if at four
months you're weighing what you should at eight,
you'll have had no choice but to add to your wardrobe.

When you do go out buying, take along a list of
essentials with the approximate price you'd be willing
to spend. Weigh any impulse item against this list.
But stay open-minded; if you see an outfit you hadn't
thought to include in your list, but which strikes you
as perfect for yourself and the demands of your life
—consider whether it could substitute for something
you did list.

YOU WILL NEED:

(As you acquire the following items, check them
off in the margins. Also make pertinent notes where
they apply.)

Day clothes. Two pairs of machine-washable maternity slacks or sport skirts in basic colors; plus
straight-cut shirts, sweaters and blouses in colors you
love; and a coat.

Job Clothes. Very useful will be a basic-color well-
cut jumper, with an assortment of sweaters, shirts
and blouses which really can be used Afterward.
These tops might also be worn with maternity slacks
or skirts. If you have a public-appearance kind of
job, add two or three daytime maternity dresses
which can double for social occasions.

Party Clothes. Be realistic in planning these—two changes should be adequate. Unless you go out a very great deal, nobody will mind seeing you in the same outfit a few times. And you'll probably be able to borrow party clothes in greater quantity and better condition than any other category. Almost everyone overbuys, and is happy to pass along, maternity dress-ups.

Remember, while shopping, that the look you want to avoid is the all-the-way-around hugeness reminiscent of the old-style maternity smock tops. That's why you should stay away from smock dresses or tops; take the A-line instead, which shows you slim and trim down the back and at the sides, with only a nice, neatly defined round Bump at the front. You get the same trim effect with one of those long, knitted button-front cardigans or vests—and the front buttons distract nicely from The Bump. Worn over a neatly cut skirt or stovepipe slacks, it gives you a slender long-legged look that tells the world you're basically a slim girl with, at the moment, a Bump.

Want to try a bit of camouflage? Over both long sweaters and A-lines, a long scarf tied softly at the neck, drifting down over The Bump, will help to blur its outlines. In jackets and coats, a good style is the wraparound. Its vagueness around the middle actually underplays The Bump's impact, though you might think it would draw attention. Dresses and jumpers with inverted pleats will give you room for expansion but lie flat enough for trimness. In general, clothes should be small in the shoulders, neat around necklines and collars, slender along thighs and legs.

In other words, accentuate the delicacy of your figure apart from The Bump, so that you look beautifully pregnant, not merely large all over.

That's why the Empire is such a wonderful shape for the lady with a Bump. The top is so delicate and skinny, and the skirt fullness starts high up so that it's not a sudden attention-getter at Bump level.

Lightweight fabrics are best. Pregnant women feel the heat more than usual, and are more subject to itchiness; so stay away from rough, heavy materials. But of course this is not the time for very thin, clinging materials either. Crisp fabrics that don't wrinkle are a good bet, as are bonded fabrics that feel pleasant inside and look shapely outside.

As for color, it's really not the main consideration. Warm colors are flattering if you're looking pale. Some think that dark colors draw less attention. Others prefer patterns—tweeds, brocades, plaids, prints—claiming that they blur your shape. Yet, my most becoming pregnancy party dress until the very end was a halter-necked drifting cloud of pure white chiffon, finished off at hemline and halter in black satin, worn over a white-crepe A-line underdress.

The best advice is: Try it on and judge. Judge style, fabric and color for the way they look on you.

Underwear. You will know—as your regular underthings begin to feel uncomfortably tight, anywhere from the fourth to the sixth month—when it's time to visit your favorite maternity shop's lingerie department. Again, don't overbuy. Most lingerie today is quick-drying and easily washed. You can get by on a minimum array.

You'll find that almost anything you wore before

you were pregnant is also available in a maternity version with expandable front panels—panties, half slips, full, culotte and bra slips, garter belts, and girdles.

You can wear your usual bra style, assuming that it's a sturdy and supportive model, in a size larger to accommodate your enlarging bosom. Stick to well-made cotton brassieres—no plastics. You can also begin to wear nursing bras if you thriftily decide you might as well get your money's worth by buying and wearing throughout pregnancy the bras you will need as a nursing mother. Your breasts are likely to leak in your latter months, so you'll want a few boxes of disposable nursing pads, too.

From about your sixth month on, your doctor may suggest that you'll feel a lot more comfortable in elastic stockings or pantihose, which soothe your legs under the new weight you're carrying. Don't worry—modern support hosiery is every bit as sensational looking as standard styles. It comes textured, patterned, colored; either fashionably opaque or quite sheer.

Shoes. If it's comfortable, wear it. Satin slippers, strappy sandals, walking clogs, boots . . . anything goes as long as you can walk in it and feel well balanced. If your feet swell—and swell they may, in pregnancy, as may your fingers—you'll need to buy new shoes a size or more larger. But don't run amok at the shoe store; your post-natal feet may very well shrink back to your old size. Consider color and style carefully so the fewest possible pairs of shoes will match the various costumes in your maternity wardrobe.

part two

the second three months

1. HOSPITAL CARE $715
    5 days at $93.00 per day for a semi-private
    room (2 in a room) $465
    Deliver...   100

chapter three

the nursery

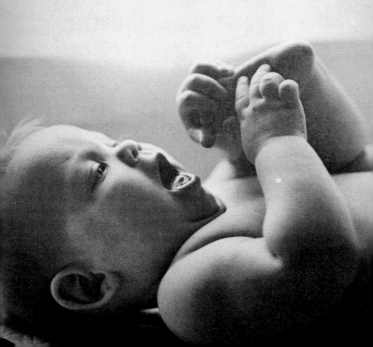

BABY'S FURNISHINGS

Maybe you've long since dealt with baby's housing problem. Maybe you decided, even before you got pregnant, exactly where you would install your future offspring. And maybe not. And if not, now! Is there room in your present apartment or house, or do you have to start hunting for a new home?

As soon as you know where baby will take up his residence—anything from a bright corner of your bedroom to a spacious nursery wing in your mansion—make a scale drawing of it.

As you hunt for nursery furniture, sketch each item you're about to buy or borrow—in scale, appropriately letter-coded, in pencil so you can erase

—into place in your room plan to make sure it will fit. Start with the essentials—the crib and the chest of drawers; then decide if and how the extra pieces will fit in.

The following rundown is all you need to assemble to start baby off in style. Unless you're so rich you just don't think about budgeting, start scouting around in your fourth month for everything you can borrow or inherit. Give the project about two months, during which time you ask everyone you know and then wait to see what is offered. Accept graciously the offers that best suit your needs and take extras, too, such as a daybed, a toy chest, anything you have room for. Record all gifts (so you remember to send out thank-you notes) on page 93, as well as the names of all donors and the items lent.

(A) CRIB. Naturally, *the* essential; baby will sleep in it for the first two to four years of his life. In fact, a full-size crib, one that measures 54" x 30" is considered a "six-year size," though in my experience almost every child graduates to a bed by the time he's four. You can also find a smaller-size crib—to fit into a smaller nursery—which has the advantage of rolling easily through doorways if you think you'll be bringing your baby up with nomadic sleeping patterns. And some cribs convert later into youth beds, saving you an extra expense in the future. Nearly all cribs today are carefully made so that the bars are no more than 3¼" apart to prevent baby's head from getting caught between them when he peeks out, and with an easily locked, deep dropside to facilitate access and yet keep him from falling out. Check to see that your selection has these features. Allowance for adjusting mattress height is also convenient, as are casters which make it easy to move the crib about. Look for strong construction (hard woods tend to hold up best), a smooth, splinter-free, durable finish, and a minimum, if any, external hardware. A plastic-coated dropside rail will keep a teething baby from eating the finish. Shop the nursery-furniture stores near you; the salespeople are generally very helpful about explaining the good points of various styles and helping you decide which is right for you. If you will be painting a hand-me-down crib, make sure your paint is lead-free.

Give as much thought to the purchase of your CRIB MATTRESS. It should be resilient yet firm to start baby on his way to healthy posture. Get the best you can; it's an important investment.

The crib is the first item to sketch into your room plan because it should be in the light, airy part of the room, but not in direct brilliant sunlight or in drafts; nor within reach of dangerously tuggable things like light cords, venetian-blind cords, and hanging pictures. Once you've found the perfect corner for the crib, the other items take their places in relation to it.

(B) CHEST OF DRAWERS. The second essential is a place to put baby's fineries—a chest of drawers or a chifforobe which combines drawers and a closet section in which you can hang garments (the latter is especially useful if you have limited closet space). Check on the construction of drawers, joints, and runners—see that they are sturdy and well-sanded so that they pose no problems to your baby when he starts crawling about. If there's someone handy at home, you could substitute built-in shelves with shutter doors or a wall-hung unit for the floor model.

Or you can look around for an old piece that needs a refinishing or paint job. (Remember: finishes and paints must be nontoxic and lead-free.)

The chest of drawers doesn't need to be waiting for the baby as the crib does; but if you plan to buy one, unless you're very tightly budgeted you might as well buy it along with the rest of your nursery furniture so that it will match. Then, too, you'll have it ready to hold not only the layette you purchase, but all the clothing you will receive as baby gifts.

(C) DRESSING TABLE. A dressing table is a help. It should stand close to the crib for your ease and comfort in transferring baby to and fro. The table should have one high shelf for diapers, so you can keep one hand on baby while the other hand reaches for a diaper; plus a lower shelf to keep changes of clothing always ready; and side pockets for baby powder, lotion, oil, cotton balls, tissues, diaper pins. If possible, the dressing table should be so placed that you can mount wall shelves (wooden or hardware) right above it to hold the extras the dressing table won't hold. And I found my table, which had a bathtub in its upper portion, a great boon during my daughter's early months. That type of dressing table saves you the expense and space for a separate baby tub—and a baby tub, small and cozy, is very helpful in making your infant's earliest bathtime experiences happy ones.

(D) DIAPER PAIL for quick disposal of soiled cloth diapers (diaper service presents this to customers at no charge); **WASTEBASKET** for used tissues, cotton balls, disposable diapers, etc.; **NURSERY HAMPER** (lined in washable vinyl) for discarded shirts and nightgowns. All of these should be placed equidistant to crib and dressing table.

(E) BASSINET. This is a pleasant extra. Psychologists say newborns are happiest in small bassinets rather than cribs that are enormous in relation to their size. But our gutsy modern babies are often too large and active for a bassinet by the time they're five or six weeks old; their squirming and turning are liable to tip over a fragile bassinet. Besides, at six weeks they begin to enjoy the larger wriggling space of a crib. So, a bassinet, while nice to have, is definitely something to borrow rather than buy. Maybe that's why so many layette shops, aware of your disinclination to invest in a brief-use bassinet, make you a gift of one with a layette purchase of seventy-five dollars or so.

If you live in a large house, where you may need to have several places for baby to nap while he follows you as you follow your chores, you will certainly want a bassinet for toting baby along. In that case, be practical: choose either one on wheels that goes everywhere in your home, or one that converts to a car bed that goes everywhere period.

Wherever you put the bassinet, keep in mind the specifications about light, air, etc. under **CRIB.**

(F) CRADLE. If you want to splurge, or if there's an heirloom in your family, this is the best bassinet of all. Rocking is very soothing to babies when they're hungry, upset or in mild discomfort, and many experts urge a return to cradles or at least to being rocked. Which brings us to—

(G) ROCKING CHAIR. Everyone seems to agree

that this is a wonderful piece of furniture for a nursery. It lets you hold baby in your arms and rock him in a gentle, soothing rhythm, and it'll be a great boon to you—it will give you a relaxing ten minutes now and then in your hectic baby-care day. Later on, the rocking chair can be a charming accessory in your child's room—an oversize toy he and his friends can ride in, a leaning-back place for grandparents while they chat with the small host. Just make sure it's a sturdy, secure model.

(H) LAMPS AND NIGHT LIGHT. Strew these about the nursery the way you would in any room—to give pleasant, useful light wherever you will need it: for dressing baby, feeding him in your rocking chair, lighting him in his crib for night viewing without throwing glare into his face. Lamps in nursery design are nice because they provide baby with a kind of toy to look at; but if you're feeling thrifty, you can paint or decal or re-shade ordinary old lamps into something just as attractive.

Try to avoid overhead light. If you must use it, try to make it indirect. You can achieve this very cheaply with a simple inverted ceiling fixture.

(I) TRAVEL STORAGE. It's helpful to keep all of baby's accouterments in his own room, so that you don't have to go dashing around the house to get him ready for excursions. Plan on a nursery corner or closet to hold such gear as a car bed, carriage, back pack, and portable crib for overnight visits.

(J) VISUAL AIDS FOR BABY. Newborns love and —psychologists say—*need* the mental stimulation of a CRIB MOBILE. They like to look around them and see things, so make the nursery walls as interesting as you can without overloading them. Put up pictures and decorations to your own family's taste, since a nursery is not only a home for baby but a magic visiting place for the rest of the family.

I once read that a baby likes to have a MIRROR in view so he can watch his fascinating self. And I've also heard mothers say that every child's room should have one BULLETIN BOARD wall—either the whole wall or a good part of it—covered in cork, felt, beaverboard or burlap, where all sorts of drawings, photographs and illustrations (later on, the child's own creations) can be taped on and taken down to suit the baby's changing interests and age.

One of the simplest and most modern visual aids is the CLEAR PLASTIC CRIB BUMPER. These bumbers are used in an infant's early weeks to protect him from banging his head against the crib bars. Unlike the traditional padded cloth bumpers, the inflated plastic bumpers allow the baby, even before it's old enough to turn over, to lie on his back and watch the world—his world, his nursery—through them.

(K) CLIMATE AIDS. Plan the right spots in your nursery for installing such optional but helpful paraphernalia as an ELECTRIC HEATER (for a winter baby, in case of heating-failure emergencies); COLD WATER HUMIDIFIER to keep the air moist in an overheated overdry winter room, especially when baby has a cold; AIR CONDITIONER or ELECTRIC FAN to be used for an older baby and only when and as your pediatrician suggests.

(L) FLOOR. Vinyl or floor tiling is perfect for

nurseries. Carpeting is lovely, but you can't just grab a mop and a handful of paper towels to whisk away baby's upchuck, or piddle, or overturned gloppy cereal, or spilled finger paints. . . . And a linoleum floor can always be scattered with small or large area rugs for cozy play corners. If you must have carpeting, at least choose a washable synthetic. In any case, don't choose a floor covering until you've first decided on the nursery's total color scheme.

(M) WALLS. Many parents begin their nursery planning with the wallpaper, but I'm a great believer in painted walls for a child's room in baby- and toddlerhood. First of all, paint can be scrubbed clean of most crayon marks; it cannot be tattered and torn by toy autos riding the walls. Paint provides a solid-tone surface on which to hang, paste or nail any pictures, plaques or objects that catch yours or baby's fancy—without worrying that these will either clash with or not show up against the wallpaper pattern. Then, too, painted walls can be done in advance in a color to suit either boy or girl, whereas the tendency to match wallpaper to sex (toy trains or stripes for a boy, ribbon bows and rosebuds for a girl) delays the process. There's also the hazard of choosing an all-purpose infant-design paper which inevitably seems too babyish by the time your child is a four-year-old individual. Finally, if you paint now, you can wallpaper later when you won't have all these other pressing expenses.

All this having been said—if your heart is set on wallpaper, go ahead. Just one last practical plea: Do think about all the pretty vinyl—meaning washable—wall coverings available today. That stunning but unwashable hand-painted paper you pine for will

drive you to distraction when your infant becomes a
crayon-wielding jam-smearing one-year-old.

(N) CURTAINS. You can choose these ahead of
time—either ready-mades or the fabric for making
them yourself—in a pattern suitable for boy or girl
(toys, fairytale, checks, plaid, gay floral) or you can
wait. Curtains can be your one deft His or Her touch
in the nursery; and if you've gotten everything else
ready, your baby's room will be pretty enough to do
without curtains for a couple of weeks and not look
barren. You can shop for these on your first post-baby
outing, or you can pre-shop by making alternate
selections and phoning in your order from the hospital. If you would like to pre-shop, when making
your selection, ask the salesperson whether the curtains (or fabric) are certain to be available about the
time you expect your baby.

The preceding rundown, A through N, is all you
need. Take your time looking. Comparison-shop as
much as you like. Try to get photos or sketches of the
items you're considering to show to your husband,
to refresh your memory before making your final
choice, and to copy into your room plan. Scotch-
tape an envelope into the inside cover of this book in
which to store them. Write down all the details too—
often you can phone in your order once you've
decided, saving you another trip to the store. Space
for these notes is provided on page 89.

By the sixth month most of your lending sources
have been heard from and you've shopped around
enough to know what you like and can afford. If you
want to have everything delivered to your home as
soon as possbile, do your ordering now. There is

often a six week to two month wait between ordering and receiving new nursery furniture. If you're buying second-hand or antique pieces, you could use this time to survey your collection and decide what needs painting or covering with Contact paper or refinishing or whatever.

Whether or not everything is physically in your nursery, now is the time to start planning in earnest. First write down the unchangeable elements in your decor. Does the nursery room already have a good linoleum vinyl floor so that you must plan everything else around its color? Do you have a good, spare carpet that would be thrifty to use? Have you always felt nursery walls *have* to be, say, pale green? Is your best friend lending you her prized maple crib whose color you find too dark but which you must return unrefinished for *her* second baby? Have you found a wonderful set of nursery furniture on sale but in a bland off-white you find too boring for words?

Look over your notes. If they add up to an effect you don't love, or if the separate elements clash, now's the time to think about a total color scheme that will blend everything together, or will counteract the effect you object to, or will change things with paint and Contact. For instance, if your crib is too dark for your taste, make everything else—other furniture, curtains, walls, floor—very light and bright. Is the floor too wishy-washy pale? Use strong colors elsewhere.

Lately, research on the psychology and learning process in infants has shown that pale pale pastels or white, while restful, are not necessarily the best for tiny babies, after all. Bright colors alert a baby's senses, stimulate him into responsiveness and mental development. If you find plain primary colors too

obvious, you can choose wonderful softened versions
like apple green, soldier blue, coral red, burnt orange,
deep pink. These stronger colors can be used on the
walls of the nursery, with the furniture in white or
complementary pastel or light wood tones. Or the
walls can be white or pastel, with the nursery fur-
nishings in the deeper shades. Buy an inexpensive
box of crayons and make rough color sketches to
give yourself an idea of color combinations. Store
them in the envelope you've attached to the inside
cover along with color cards of furniture- and wall-
paint * colors or wallpaper swatches.

The paint should be washable. Two coats will en-
sure that you can sponge away any smudges the
toddler thinks to contribute to his walls. Even so,
you may have to touch up scoured-off paint at the
scene of his more enterprising messes. Keep a large,
tightly closed canful of your nursery paint to repair
such future disasters.

Do your painting—or have it done—in the seventh
month. Or make arrangements now to have all this
done between the day the baby is born and the day
you come home from the hospital. Have your boy-
choice and girl-choice colors all set in writing for
the painters so they'll know just how to proceed on
a go-ahead phone call from you or Daddy on birth
day. (You should anticipate, however, that you'll
have a problem about where to put baby for a couple
of days until the paint smell is all gone.)

---

* Make sure all paints are non-toxic and without a lead base. If your
nursery is in an older building and you suspect that previous coats
of paint *were* lead-base, cover the walls thoroughly with two coats
of non-lead-base paint. Babies have a way of peeling paint right off
anything and eating it.

BABY'S TRAVEL GEAR

By the time your baby is three weeks old, he'll be ready to cut out from his nursery, to go places and do things. About the seventh month of pregnancy, then, you ought to be deciding what these places and things will be and what equipment you'll need.

First, probably, a baby carriage. But which kind? There's a carriage style for just about every way of life there is. A big, heavy Rolls Royce of a carriage from England—warm because it's so solidly built, smooth-riding because of its excellent springs, wonderful for cold climates and bumpy walking paths. But bulky. And expensive.

Then there are compromise versions of the same idea—that is, big, strong, hard-sided carriages for rugged weather or terrain, but less imposing and less expensive than the poshest English models. There are also soft, light carriages with the advantages of easy handling and small storage requirements. Fold-up carriages for easy transportability. Carriages that convert quickly into car beds.

There are also car beds per se. And travel cribs for overnight visits. And travel playpens. And, in recent years, all sorts of back- or front-packs for strapping baby to *you* and walking him to your destination—a cozy idea young Americans have adopted from Indians and other non-urban, non-vehicular peoples.

Decide on your needs, look at everything in your favorite infant's stores, and keep your eyes open for possible lenders. You might want to add some travel items to your Rich Uncle Page.

THE LAYETTE

About the same time that you're painting and fixing up your nursery, you should order your layette.

What color should it be? When should you have it delivered to your home? If you want a layette in white or yellow or green for your baby, girl or boy, you can have it sent home immediately and arrange everything in your nursery shelves and drawers so it's waiting neatly for baby's homecoming. But if you're a traditionalist and want to have the appropriate pink or blue, infants' shops routinely take early orders, get everything ready, and send a pink or blue or whatever layette to your home within hours of your phone call from the hospital.*

If possible, buy all or at least most of your layette at one store. Not only is your bookkeeping less complicated that way, but the store will often make you a gift of some lovely extra with the purchase of a large layette.

Most authorities agree pretty much on what the newborn's wardrobe and linens should include. The following lists may be more or less generous than some you will see, but you needn't follow them slavishly. These lists are simply the ones I found adequate (as confirmed by my favorite maternity nurse, herself the mother of two toddlers) for starting my own motherly existence with a clean supply of clothes and sheets always on hand, and without spending my whole day at the washing machine. If you can launder more often, buy less. If you want to decrease your laundry chores, you may want to

* Record all pertinent information in the space provided for it on page 89.

increase the quantities I suggest. You can always
order by telephone whatever additional items you
find you need after your laundry routines are set during baby's first couple of weeks. But don't overdo
it—infants outgrow their clothes very quickly. And
bear in mind that your own layette purchases will
probably be supplemented by small gifts brought by
friends on their introductory visits to baby. Not to
speak of hand-me-downs in good condition, offered
to you by the other young mothers in your crowd.

As you purchase your layette, check off the items
on the lists.

If you plan to have your layette delivered after the
birth of your baby, record all the information you will
need on page 89.

Baby's Wardrobe

12 cotton-knit gowns. The kind that don't open down
the front make diaper-changing a bit more tricky,
but they're more snug for winter babies.

6 cotton-knit kimonos or robes. To go over the
gowns for extra warmth; or to be worn alone, without gowns, in hot weather.

6 cotton-knit undershirts with snaps for easy
changing.

6 pairs waterproof pants

6 pairs newborn-size socks
newborn-style and/or soft shoes or booties for a
winter baby

8 cotton-flannel receiving blankets. To wrap around
baby in a dozen different situations during the day.

2 sweaters. For outings; cotton for summer, wool or Orlon for winter.

2 hats

1 bunting or carriage suit or equivalent. For any baby except one born in hottest midsummer.

4 stretch-terrycloth jump suits. Also known as creepers. Baby won't start wearing these until he's about 2 months old and kicking too much to stay immobile and wrapped in his gown and receiving blanket. But buy four of them along with the rest of your layette so you're sure to have a few on hand when baby is ready for them. You'll probably need more than four, but wait and see if you receive extras as gifts. If not, phone-order what you need.

4 sunsuits. To augment or substitute for creepers for a baby who'll be two to four months old in midsummer. However, if your house is air-conditioned, sunsuits are not necessarily a good idea.

3 diaper sets. Pretty costumes for showing off a newborn to his visitors. Quantity depends on how many visitors you expect. I find tiny babies pretty enough without these costumes—just in their dainty gowns and blankets—but more clothes-conscious mothers will love them.

1 christening gown.

Clothing to bear in mind for later. Zipper-front blanket-cloth jump suit for sleeping, snow suits, bathrobes, little dresses and suits, extra sweaters and jackets. . . . You will need all these in the coming months. But don't buy them now. First of all, you will receive many as gifts. Second, if you wait to buy them, you'll be able to select clothes to suit the individual your infant has become. And, finally, why crowd your nursery drawers now with things you won't need for several months?

Diapers

Diaper service will probably cost you about two hundred and fifty dollars for baby's first year. From the hospital you or someone else can call a company to institute delivery for the day you expect to be home. They generally respond on twenty-four hours' notice and advise you on quantities to order. Choose a company ahead of time (on friends' recommendations) and note the information on page 84.

In addition, though, you should always have at least a dozen of your own cloth diapers—or a box or two of disposable ones—on hand to supplement the service. You'll want them around for the baby, but also to use over your shoulder for baby's spitting up.

If you'd rather home-launder diapers, buy three or four dozen, plus the special diaper laundry products your pediatrician recommends to soak out the bacteria that cause diaper rash in infants. You can buy these items ahead, or have someone pick them up after you give birth.

If you prefer disposable diapers—they're getting better all the time—you'll need three boxes to start, with constant replenishing. You can buy disposables ahead if you like, but it's just as easy to buy them later. They will probably cost you about two hundred and fifty dollars for baby's first year.

And don't forget diaper pins. And a diaper bag for outings.   *Continued on page 97*

❧ *Nine* *Months of* *Notes* ❧

Here are a number of lists that will be a real help at this busy time. Use the Pregnancy Calendar to schedule your days and keep track of appointments and errands. Consider the suggestions of things to do each month as a guide; alter them to suit your needs. Space is also provided for important addresses and phone numbers, for recording expenses and possible baby names, for keeping track of borrowed things that have to be returned and gifts that have to be acknowledged. A birth announcement list, a nursery planning list, a record of agencies and businesses whose services you've hired—everything in one place. You'll find these lists very handy and you'll certainly enjoy looking through them again, when all has calmed down, when your son or your daughter is the only reality, and having been pregnant a memory far in the past.

Pregnancy Calendar

MONTH 1

Choose obstetrician and hospital
Consult your health-insurance policy
Enter all doctor appointments

Date	Day	Time	Appointments & Things to do
9	14	2.00	Dr. Jeffries - Greenbelt 552-3000 937-0121 Beltsville

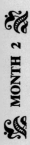

MONTH 2

Make dentist appointments
Estimate your expenses
Enter all doctor appointments

Date	Day	Time	Appointments & Things to do
			....
			....
			....
			....
			....
			....
			....
			....

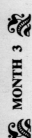

MONTH 3

Interview newborn nurse candidates
Enter all doctor appointments

Date Day Time Appointments & Things to do

....

....

....

....

....

....

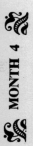

🐾 MONTH 4 🐾

Start planning the nursery
Shop for baby furniture
Ask around for maternity clothes
Enter all doctor appointments

Date   Day   Time   Appointments & Things to do

....

....

....

....

....

....

....

69

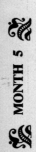

MONTH 5

Register for parenthood class
Register for natural childbirth class
Enter all doctor appointments

Date	Day	Time	Appointments & Things to do

Date   Day   Time   Appointments & Things to do

71

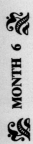

🐾 MONTH 6 🐾

Arrange for delivery of nursery furniture
Start planning baby's layette
Shop for baby's travel gear
Shop for necessary maternity clothes
Enter all doctor appointments

Date   Day   Time   Appointments & Things to do

....

....

....

....

....

....

....

Date   Day   Time   Appointments & Things to do

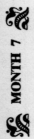

MONTH 7

Paint the nursery
Order baby's layette
Choose a diaper service
See a printer about birth announcements
Complete birth announcement list
Make preparations for religious ceremonies
Enter all doctor appointments

Date	Day	Time	Appointments & Things to do

74

Date	Day	Time	Appointments & Things to do

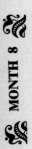

❧ MONTH 8 ❧

Start natural childbirth class
Choose godparents
Choose a pediatrician
Enter all doctor appointments

Date   Day   Time   Appointments & Things to do

....

....

....

....

....

....

Date   Day   Time   Appointments & Things to do

77

✒ MONTH 9 ✒

Pack your hospital suitcase
Double-check plans for getting to the hospital
Get your house in order
Enter all doctor appointments

Date	Day	Time	Appointments & Things to do

Date   Day   Time   Appointments & Things to do

....

....

....

....

....

....

....

....

....

....

....

....

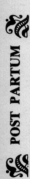

POST PARTUM

Call or have someone else call all the people listed on page 137, and those whose names are asterisked on the Birth Announcement list. Finish filling in Chores for the New Father.

Date	Day	Time	Appointments & Things to do
			....
			....
			....
			....
			....
			....
			....

Date   Day   Time   Appointments & Things to do

81

🌿 Important Addresses and Phone Numbers 🌿

Obstetrician

Address

Phone

Hospital

Address

Phone

Dentist

Address

Phone

Pediatrician

Address

Phone

Name

Address

Phone

Name

Address

Phone

Name

Address

Phone

Name

Address

Phone

Name

Address

Phone

Name

Address

Phone

Name

Address

Phone

Name

Address

Phone

Name

Address

Phone

Name

Address

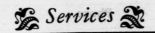

Services

DIAPER SERVICE

Name   Phone   Comments

TAXI SERVICE

Name   Phone   Comments

NURSE EMPLOYMENT AGENCIES

Name   Phone   Comments

NURSE OR HOUSEKEEPER CANDIDATES

Name   Phone   Comments
                        home and job

PAINTER OR PAPERHANGER

Name	Phone	Agreed price

BIRTH ANNOUNCEMENTS

Printer's name	Phone	Comments

🦌 Expenses 🦌

Unless you're very wealthy, you'll want to arrive at an estimate of your expenses so you can work out a budget, or in some way figure out how much money you are going to need and where it's going to come from. Record the expenses you and your doctor foresee, and the estimates you get from the hospital. You'll find the approximate figures for many of the expenses that fall under Infant's Needs and Personal Expenses throughout the book. Space has been provided for you to add additional expenses as you encounter them.

When you start paying your bills, enter your actual figures in the column next to the estimated. You'll want to keep track of these figures for your own record and for tax purposes. Check off those that can be taken off on your taxes in the column labeled tax deductible.

	estimated cost	actual cost	tax deductible
HOSPITAL CARE			
private room	....	....	....
semi-private room	....	....	....
ward	....	....	....
delivery room charge	....	....	....
nursery charge	....	....	....
circumcision set-up	....	....	....
anaesthesia	....	....	....
MEDICAL CARE			
obstetrician	....	....	....
circumcision fee	....	....	....
pediatrician fee	....	....	....

	estimated cost	actual cost	tax deductible
dentist			
newborn nurse			
INFANT'S NEEDS			
basic layette			
diaper service			
linens			
crib			
chest of drawers			
dressing table			
baby carriage			
playpen			

PERSONAL EXPENSES	estimated cost	actual cost	tax deductible
maternity clothes			
parenthood class			
natural childbirth class			
religious ceremony fee			
housekeeper			
transportation			
interest on loans			
TOTAL EXPENSE			
LESS INSURANCE COVERAGE			
TOTAL EXPENSE			

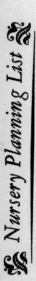

꩜ Nursery Planning List ꩜

If you plan to have nursery fittings and layette delivered after the birth of your baby, you should list all the information you will need here. When your baby arrives, alert the shops (let them know your final color decisions) and the merchandise will be sent right away.

Item	Store	Salesperson	Phone	Sales-slip number	Price	Date bought

Item	Store	Salesperson	Phone	Sales-slip number	Price	Date bought

Borrowed Things

During your pregnancy, and for your baby's first few months, you'll need many short-use items. Try to save on these expenses by borrowing as many as you can from previously pregnant friends and relatives. Ask around for maternity clothes, baby clothes, and furniture for the nursery. Keep this list of what belongs to whom so that when you're through with the items you can return them to their rightful owners.

Item	Lent by	Address	Phone number	Comments

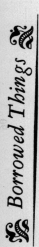

Naming Your Baby

BOYS			GIRLS		
Name	Middle Name	Surname	Name	Middle Name	Surname

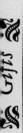

Gifts

It'll be better than Christmas as all the lovely gifts come in for you and your baby. But if you don't keep up with your Thank-you Notes, the festivity of it all will turn into a mere chore. Try to send off a short appreciative note whenever you receive a gift instead of letting them pile up for some mythical day you've earmarked for note writing. With your new baby at home, an unharried day will be long in coming.

As you open each gift, record the item you receive and the names of the people who have sent it so you don't end up thanking the wrong friend for the wrong gift. Whenever possible, enter the store from which the gift came so you can exchange duplicate items.

Gift	From (name & address)	Store	Date received	Date acknowledged

Gift	From (name & address)	Store	Date received	Date acknowledged

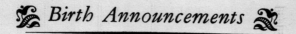

Birth Announcements

Start compiling this list, at your leisure, early in your pregnancy, giving yourself time to think of everyone and to check on addresses. Place an asterisk next to the names of those people who should be called from the hospital with the Arrival news.

Name	Address	Phone

Name	Address	Phone

Bed Linens

4 fitted bassinet sheets. If you're using a bassinet.
Standard pillowcases are a good substitute.

6 fitted crib sheets. Cotton-knit no-iron sheets are
pleasant for baby, easy-to-launder for you. Sheets
printed with delicate floral or toy motifs give baby
something interesting to look at during his earliest
weeks.

6 under-sheet crib-size quilted pads.

4 crib-size waterproof flannelized pads.

2 crib blankets or quilts.

Bath Linens

6 washcloths.

6 baby-size bath towels. With one corner shaped
as a hood for his little damp head.

1 Mommy-size terrycloth bathing apron, with pockets for you.

Carriage Linens

4 fitted carriage sheets. Again, cotton-knit no-iron
ones are nice.

1 carriage pillow.

2 carriage pillowcases.

1 carriage cover.

Elaborate carriage covers and pillowcases are
among the most popular baby gifts. So keep your own
purchases of these items to minimum until you see

what you receive. Should you find yourself short, you
can always order additions by phone.

Shopping for twins. Don't worry. Just buy a single
layette. And if you turn out to be doubly blessed,
phone your infants' shop—most stores make it a
happy custom to send you two of everything at no
additional charge.

RICH UNCLE PAGE

Within baby's first few months you will already
begin to need—or anyway want—a staggering ware-
houseful of equipment for that one tiny creature.
Have your answers ready when your rich uncle
chucks you under the chin and asks you what he can
give the little darling? Or, on a more prosaic level,
start lining up borrowing prospects as you did with
your basic nursery. If the following list doesn't give
you enough ideas, you can always look around your
local nursery shops for the newest inventions in baby-
consumerdom. Meantime, check off the items here
as they're either purchased or promised.

ITEM	SOURCE
Eating Table or Highchair	
Carriage	
Playpen	
Travel Bed or Seat	
Reclining Seat	
Baby Swing	
Walker	
Toy Chest	
Daybed	

ITEM	SOURCE
Stroller	
Matched Set of French Provincial Nursery Furniture	
Extra Tables	
Extra Chairs	
Door-Guard Fences	
Window Bars	
Extra Telephone Extension for Nursery	

chapter four

preparing for birth

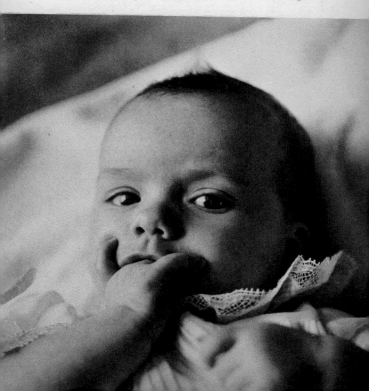

NATURAL CHILDBIRTH CLASS

Regardless of whether or not you're sure about natural childbirth, you should take a course. There's something about the training that, through knowledge, lessens your fears; through exercise, prepares your muscles; through giving you things to do during labor and delivery, actually takes your mind off waiting for that pain you always heard about. . . . The techniques, by the way, are much easier than you ever expected. You'll learn them quickly and get good at them with no trouble.

And it's good for you to take a course. You *can* merely read the right books and practice at home with or without your husband, but it's nicer to join a class. You'll be with a group of other women who have the right attitude—wanting to help themselves and believing they can—that will rub off on you. It did on me.

Besides, in a class you'll have the benefit of a trained natural childbirth coach advising you on how you're doing and offering you individual helpful tips. It's quite inexpensive; the most reputable private coaches in high-cost New York City charge between thirty and fifty dollars for the entire six-session course, and hospitals ask from fifteen to forty dollars.

This book will not describe the natural childbirth techniques; your class will teach you everything you need to know. What does follow is a timetable for going out and training yourself, unless you have a very good reason not to. And remember—cowardice, far from stopping you, should be your motivation.

In choosing your obstetrician in your first month, make sure he'll cooperate with you in letting you use natural childbirth techniques. I find it hard to believe, but I've been told that some doctors will not cooperate. Your doctor won't train you, but he will cooperate with you during labor and delivery while you employ your training.

In your fourth month, start asking around about classes—ask your doctor and natural childbirth enthusiasts among your friends for a good class to take. If your hospital gives such a course, ask the office to sign you up as early as necessary. Classes usually start in the eighth month, but are so popular they're usually filled far ahead. Register as soon as you can. If none of these sources has any information for you, write to the American Society for Psychoprophylaxis, 7 West 96th Street, New York, N.Y. 10025, or to the International Childbirth Education Association, Inc., 11040 West Bluemound Road, Milwaukee, Wisconsin 53226 for the name of a natural childbirth center near you.

You start classes toward the end of the seventh month or at the beginning of the eighth. Follow your exercise routine like a good girl, exactly as your teacher tells you to do. It doesn't take much time, it's easy, and it's good for your health and baby's. Keep track of your class schedule on the Pregnancy Calendar.

When it's time to leave for the hospital, in addition to your hospital suitcase, you natural childbirth trainees will need a special kit. Get it ready at the same time as you prepare your suitcase. Use a shaving kit or zippered make-up bag; either is small enough to keep with you as you go from your hospital's admitting office to the labor room. As you can see, the kit contains only a few things to keep you cool, comfortable and in command as you do the job you've been training for.

Lemon candies, on the sour side. These are good thirst-quenchers to suck on during labor and they don't fill you up as water does.

Talcum in a shaker-top box or a sponge or washcloth to be kept moist by husband or nurse. Any of these will keep you feeling cool and comfortable.

Stopwatch with second hand.

Pad and pencil. Watch and writing materials are for timing contractions—a task that really helps you feel in command.

PARENTHOOD CLASS

You didn't realize, did you?, that getting ready to have a child involves becoming a schoolgirl again yourself. Not only are you taking natural childbirth classes—I hope—but you ought to think, too, about signing up for lessons in parenthood. You and your husband both.

Your doctor is taking excellent care of you, and giving you all the important advice on caring for yourself and your baby-to-be in there. But if he's like most busy modern doctors, his waiting room is so jammed on your visits he doesn't have time to answer all your curiosity questions. Besides, he knows that if you really care, you'll enroll for an inexpensive course—ten or fifteen dollars at a hospital, perhaps even free at a community center. You should start early in the seventh month, so you have time to complete the entire curriculum.

Such a course consists of a one- or two-hour session once a week, for six to twelve weeks, sometimes for expectant mothers only but often for fathers too. They teach you about all the changes and fascinating developments inside you. They sometimes give you enough exercise and posture training so you can dispense with extra exercise classes. They explain *why* you should eat *what;* reassure you about the toughness and endurance of the fetus so you don't go around on tippy-toe in misinformed, unfounded fear of hurting "it"; help you decide on breast-feeding versus bottle-feeding; teach you the proper health and figure care for yourself after delivery; and most reassuring of all with a first baby, train you in the proper care and treatment of "it" once it's born.

If you're not planning to employ a newborn nurse, this sort of baby training will be invaluable for you and your husband—unless you're an old hand. If your local hospital or community center doesn't have such a course, and your doctor can't recommend one, phone your local Red Cross, or Visiting Nurse Association, or Public Health Office for information. Or write to the Maternity Center Association, 48 East 92nd Street, New York, N.Y. 10028.

PREPARATION FOR BREAST-FEEDING

Probably you already have an emotional preference for either bottle- or breast-feeding, based on your own temperament and your theories about child-rearing. And you could do a lot worse than simply following your instincts in this matter. Because if you do what you consider wise and pleasant, you'll be happier—which, of course, means your baby will be happy too.

But you should not get yourself locked into either choice. For instance, you may be eager to breast-feed but your milk flow may prove insufficient, or other physical factors may prevent you, or your way of life may be too hectic to permit you to keep to a nursing schedule.

Nowadays there's a great body of scientific opinion that any new mother, given the proper medical and emotional encouragement, can have a sufficient milk flow for breast-feeding—and that every baby will benefit psychologically and physically from being breastfed. But there is an equally strong medical opinion that many mothers *and* their babies are better off with bottle feedings.

Near the end of your pregnancy you and your husband should talk frankly about which method you prefer. *His* preferences come into this a great deal, since a nursing mother's time is often neither her own nor her husband's. The two of you should know exactly what breast-feeding entails and agree on it beforehand. Get your doctor's opinion too, and learn what you can in your parenthood class. And both parents will be better equipped to decide if both do some reading on the subject.

ROOMING-IN

To room-in or not to room-in, that is the question. As with the choice between breast-feeding and bottles, you should follow your instinct but learn what you can in parenthood class. Stay open-minded because even if you opt for rooming-in now, after delivery you and your doctor may feel that you should either delay rooming-in for a couple of days or dispense with it entirely.

Rooming-in means, of course, that the day after delivery the baby comes to live in the mother's hospital room rather than in the general nursery. With the nurses' supervision, she feeds him, cuddles him, diapers him, has him sleep alongside her—and in all ways starts her maternal life right in the hospital. This has the advantage of easing her into the joys and jobs of motherhood gradually, while the built-in aids and baby-sitters of the hospital staff are still hovering near, instead of thrusting her suddenly into her new role when she arrives home.

The father benefits too. With rooming-in he need only wash his hands and put on a hospital gown, and he can spend his visiting hours with you *and* baby in your room. He can hold his child and even diaper it, instead of just smiling at it through a glass window.

If this arrangement sounds like what you want, be sure your hospital provides it. Not all do.

But don't think you're a cold-hearted mother if you'd rather not have rooming-in. Even without it, you'll see your baby often for cuddling and feeding visits. At most, you'll probably be postponing full-time motherhood only three or four days—until you and your baby go home together. And since a new-born sleeps during most of its first days, and you will want to be napping a lot too, you won't be missing all that much if you do your sleeping in separate places—you in your room, baby in the general nursery. There is no medical evidence at all that rooming-in babies are in any way emotionally healthier later on.

Many new mothers feel that they're going home to a pretty heavy if joyous load of responsibility. They feel that they're doing the baby more good by using their hospital stay for thorough rest and preparation for the tiring weeks ahead, by providing him with an unfrazzled mother during his first weeks at home.

You know yourself. Decide which set of advantages best suits *you*. Then answer the question.

FATHER HOUR

Even if you don't choose rooming-in, your husband can still get to know his new baby if your hospital provides a Father Hour arrangement. This is just what it says: an hour, usually in the evening, reserved especially for new fathers. Starting on the day after birth, the baby is wheeled into your room, where your husband is waiting in a sterile hospital gown. For the whole hour, under the helpful prompting of a nurse, daddy does the cuddling, the bottle-feeding, burping, diapering when necessary. For the typical baby-shy male, this is a marvelous introductory offer. Look into it.

part three

the last three months

chapter five
the festive formalities

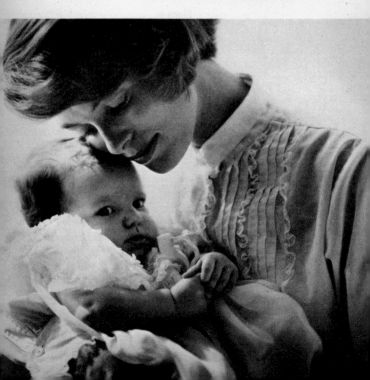

NAMING THE BABY

In every culture, throughout history and all over the world, giving birth to a baby is one of the great milestones in anyone's life. As such, it is always marked with certain rituals. One of the most enjoyable and informal is the naming of the baby. As we have seen, there are a number of important practical questions to consider early in your pregnancy. But most expectant parents, before they give a thought to anything practical, fall into a universal happy obsession the moment they learn they're going to have a baby: what to call "it"?

There's a lot of tried and true advice on the question. If you have a simple, one- or two-syllable

surname, give the baby (especially a girl) a lilting
three- or four-syllable first name. Conversely, if you
have a complicated multi-syllable surname, choose
a simple one- or two-syllable first name. Some examples: Miranda Hunt, John Hammersmith, David
Eisenhower.

There are two schools of thought on the nation-
ality of names. Some people feel that the first and
last names should match (Carmen Villanova, for
instance). Others like a contrast between the two
(Jose Hannigan, say).

Then there is the question of vowels. If the surname begins with a vowel, it's a little unmellifous to
have the first name end with one: Teresa Anderson.
The same holds for consonants: Ralph Barnes . . .
Millicent Taylor. Although some consonants do link
up harmoniously: Brian Tucker.

There are religious considerations. Orthodox Jews
are forbidden to name children for relatives still
living. Certain Protestant sects lean toward Old
Testament names. Catholics like saints' names.

And it's fun to name children for a political, lit-
erary, theatrical, sports or other celebrity you particularly admire.

But whatever name you choose, for whatever of
the above dictates of taste or belief, remember that
you are not only naming a baby—you are giving a
person an identification for life. Some names are
adorable for infants, but an embarrassment down
through the years. This is a mistake more often visited
on girls than on boys; your little pink Didi, for instance, may grow up to be a six-feet-tall lady physics
professor.

Middle names come in handy here. Since you
can't foresee the kind of adult lurking in your un-

born baby, give him an option now, to be redeemed at his maturity. That is, provide him with a middle name as opposite in aura as possible to his first name. Then let him decide in adulthood which suits him best. Be careful that your baby's initials won't cause him or her any embarrassment as might the initials formed by the names Francis Allen Garvey, or Diane Ursula Dickens, or Peter Issac Golden.

Don't worry about providing a suitable name for your child's infancy. Just dub him nobly and well, and babyhood will take care of itself. Even a Winthrop gets called Winnie-pooh at kitchy-koo age. The Queen of England, so aptly and regally known as Elizabeth to us now, was the cuddly "Lilybet" in her first years. You, too, will find kissy nicknames for your Alexandra (Sansie?) or Sebastian (Bassie?) plus a dozen nuzzling little endearment-names: Honey Doll, Baby Love, Boysie, Dollsie, Lambsie. . . . You'd be surprised at what you'll find yourself murmuring into a tiny shoulder soon!

And yet one friend of mine—a father—says his unfailing rule for naming a child is to insert the name in the following sentence, to be imagined called through a window: "Mrs. Jones, can _____ come out and play now?" Does it sound all right? Good.

I have an addition, though. After the name passes my friend's test, also make sure it passes this one: The child is now a grown man or woman, successfully pursuing a career. He or she is being discussed by the heads of the company. Insert the name into the following sentence. "Do you think _____ is capable of taking over the new department?"

And while we're at it, try the name in this sentence: "I want to marry you, _____." The way things are going, this sentence can be spoken to either sex. Women's liberation will be long completed by the time your bouncing baby boy is old enough to be proposed to by a self-possessed girl of the future.

Speaking of Women's Lib, a girl born now may very well retain even after marriage what we now call her "maiden name." So when you enter the names you're considering in the space provided for them on page 92, always attach your surname—for girls too.

BIRTH ANNOUNCEMENTS

In our society, the sending of birth announcements is common practice. These usually go out within the baby's first week or two, but you should get to your mailing list long before that. In your seventh month, start to cull names from your personal address book and your Christmas-card list. Invite the soon-to-be grandparents to make their own additions. Give yourself plenty of time to think of every name as a yardstick for deciding how many announcements to order. List the names in the space provided for them on page 95 for your own reference and for any volunteer envelope addressers. Put bright red asterisks (plus phone numbers) next to the names of those special friends and relatives who should be telephoned with the Arrival news.

If you want to send specially printed announcements, discuss choices with your local printer. He has available everything from casual "fun" announcements to elegant traditional ones. Settle on the style and price you want, and arrange with him the procedure for phoning in the exact details to be filled in after the birth. Order at least an extra dozen announcements since there are bound to be a few last-minute additions to your list. Generally the printer has the announcements ready for you within one week of your phone call from the hospital. Record all the information you will need on page 85.

Many hospitals, especially large ones, have their own facilities for printing up birth announcements. They take your order as soon as you know the baby's name and have the cards ready for you well before you leave the hospital. It's very convenient if you want to dispense with print-shop discussions. If you are interested, you should phone your hospital admitting office and ask whether they offer this service.

Also available are store-bought birth announcements on which you fill in the salient details after the birth of your baby. If you prefer these (they are less expensive), go shopping with your husband and decide together on the card you both like. Have "It's a Girl!" and "It's a Boy!" alternates staked out. Then your husband can just pick up the appropriate one when the time comes.

Or you might like to make your own announcements, as more and more young parents enjoy doing, or at least compose your own message. In that case shop ahead in the same way for the supplies or note paper you'll need. And keep in mind that the announcement should certainly include the following information: your name and your husband's, the baby's full name, whether it's a daughter or a son, the correct birth date, since many recipients will immediately transfer this to their birthday-record books. Optional information can include the exact hour and minute of the baby's arrival, its weight, and older brothers' and sisters' names.

THANK-YOU NOTES

As the birth announcements go out, gifts will start to come in. You can thank the givers either with commercial thank-you cards (to which you can add a simple personal reference to the particular gift) or with handwritten notes on any sort of stationery you like—so-called "informals" with your name printed on them, monogrammed note paper, unmarked but appropriately tinted sheets, anything.

By your ninth month, be sure you either have a good supply of this kind of stationery on hand or your husband knows where to pick it up for you on short notice so you'll have enough to keep up with your thank-you's as gifts arrive. If you wait to order your stationery *after* the baby arrives, you'll find yourself having to write your notes all at once, during days filled with feedings and diaper-changing.

Enter each gift as you unwrap it on page 93. Otherwise you may forget whom to thank for what.

RELIGIOUS CEREMONIES

Depending on your religious practice, there will be for many Christians a christening or baptismal ceremony, and for many Jews the religious circumcision rites (*Brith*) for a boy. In your seventh month, you should confer with your clergyman or rabbi about the religious ceremonies you will want and the preparations you will have to make.

GODPARENTS

Godparents are, literally, the spiritual sponsors of their godchild. That is, they are supposed to be his

examples of the proper religious life, and responsible
for his religious training if his own parents should
die. So, naturally, you want to choose godparents
who belong to your faith and whom you consider
reliable in these matters. Choose from among your
close friends, people who are likely to maintain a
special interest in your child. Relatives are not
usually asked to be godparents—the traditional
thinking being that they would watch over the child
anyway, but that a friend in becoming a godparent
increases the child's family.

Different religions and sects have different rules
about the number of godparents a child should have,
and there are equally varying traditions about the
godparents' attendance at christenings and the like.
Discuss all this thoroughly with your clergyman. And
consult any standard etiquette book for the cere-
monial fine points.

The traditional etiquette, by the way, is to ask
friends to serve as godparents immediately after the
child's birth. But you'd better have it arranged pro-
visionally beforehand.

PEDIATRICIAN

And your pediatrician will be, for over a decade,
the health sponsor of your child. As with godparents,
you don't really need to choose a pediatrician until
after birth, but it's just as well to have that settled
ahead too. Your obstetrician will recommend someone for you. Or you may already know of a pediatrician you'd feel secure with. In either case, you
normally have your first pediatrician appointment
for when the baby is three weeks old. If necessary,
your obstetrician will call in the pediatrician earlier.

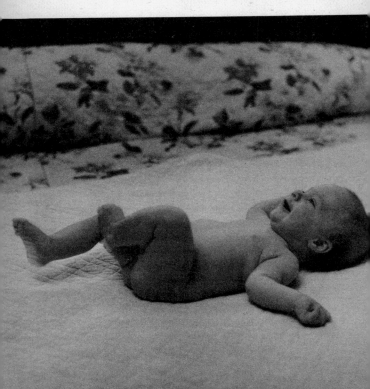

chapter six

hospital preparations

YOUR HOSPITAL SUITCASE

Reread the introduction to this book, and take it as a warning: Get your suitcase packed early, or you may find yourself depending on your husband to sniff out your tucked-away hospital essentials. Because of my own experience I *know* every woman should pack that bag the moment she enters the ninth month, sooner if her doctor feels there's any chance the baby might be premature.

Of course you may still get caught, if your pregnancy is the rare one that culminates in an extremely, unexpectedly premature birth. But in that case— as with all the advised schedules and lists in this book—though you may not have time to implement your plans, at least everything is written down in one easy-to-find place for you or someone else to work from, quickly.

Perhaps as early as your sixth month you might Scotch-tape a packing list to the inside lid of the suitcase you'll be taking to the hospital. Check off the items on the following list that you will want, then copy them onto the list you will tape to your suitcase. Now put it away until the time comes to pack. If that should prove to be a rush occasion, or if your husband ends up having to pack for you as mine did, at least there'll be a complete guide all ready.

As for the suitcase itself . . . Before you tape your list to it, first assemble the contents, then judge which piece of luggage from your present supply will accommodate it all most compactly. If you don't have the right luggage, scout around for lenders. No luck? Buy, with an eye to future usefulness.

WHAT TO BRING

This book. For all the lists you'll need for hospital chores and numbers you may want to call.

Personal phone book. For other numbers you may want to call.

Birth announcements. If you've bought them in advance.

Thank-you stationery. To acknowledge early gifts from the leisure of your hospital room.

Stamps, ballpoint pen, mechanical pencil.

1 book, 1 magazine. Your husband can bring you more as you need them; don't overload your suitcase now.

Needlework or **knitting** if that, rather than reading, is your bag. But nothing too bulky—again, your husband can bring you more later.

Nail polish, and **manicure tools.**

Make-up, lotions, deodorant, special soap, perfume, powder—in a **plastic bag** or **zippered kit,** if you'll need to carry your make-up things to a bathroom mirror.

Make-up mirror. For making-up in comfort at your bed.

Tweezer.

Eyeglasses or **contacts.**

Shower cap.

Toothbrush and **toothpaste.**

Hairbrush and **comb, bobby pins, hairpins, rollers, curlers** (but not electric).

Tissues and/or **handkerchiefs, cotton balls,** if you use them for make-up and face cleansing.

Housecoat. Something loose and easy and attractive for strolling the hospital corridors to visit your baby or any friends you may have made among the other new mothers.

Slippers. Backless scuffs are easy to slip into if you don't feel like bending over yet, and they leave room for your feet which may still be a bit pregnancy-swollen. Any heel height you're comfortable in is all right, except after a Caesarean delivery, when high heels are not a good idea.

Bed jacket. There's nothing like a smashing bed jacket for sitting up and receiving visitors, as you will be doing. I found myself trying to look snappy in my bunched-up housecoat and it just wasn't the same thing at all! Get yourself a bed jacket—it's a lifetime investment. You can always put it away for future pregnancies or even for staying in bed with a cold.

Nightgowns. For the normal four- to five-day childbirth stay, three washable gowns will do nicely. For an eight- to ten-day stay after a Caesarean, pack five because you may not want to wash that often.

But "washable" does not necessarily mean nylon if you find nylon hot or if it's summertime; you may be happier with cool no-iron cotton or dacron-and-cotton—they're just as washable. And you will want to wash your gowns. It's hot, resting in bed a lot, and it's refreshing to change your gown. Besides, during your entire hospital stay (and after) you will have menstrual-type bleeding, and your gowns may stain. For that reason, short gowns are better than long (less likely to stain); and pajamas or babydolls are not too great because the pants will stain (as well as make the nurses' periodic examinations of you a little more difficult).

Low-cut gowns are pleasant because they're cool. And certainly if you plan to breast-feed you want gowns that either open in front or slip easily off your shoulders. On the other hand, if you're not going to nurse your baby you may be wearing a binder to help slow down your milk production; and then you'll want attractively styled high-neckline gowns to cover the binder.

So much for practicalities. Almost as important: pack gowns that you consider madly flattering, in heavenly colors. The day after delivery, after months of pushing that Bump ahead of her, almost every woman alive feels the urge to prove she's back in competition. And a maternity floor is jumping with other good-looking young women, and nice doctors, and visitors, and most of all your husband who can stop telling you now that a woman is her most beautiful in the advanced stages of pregnancy!

Panties. Many women feel naked without these and pack a full supply for the hospital. Well, don't. You really won't be able to wear them until the third day after birth, when the bleeding wanes. Then, four or five washable pairs will be quite enough; knit cotton is cooler than nylon for long rests in bed. A good idea is to pack only your baggy old maternity panties and use them for the last time in the hospital. When they stain, don't bother to wash them; just throw them out. Then, back home, you can start your post-Bump life with lovely new underthings.

Bras. Even if you're usually a bra-less type, every new mother should wear a bra all the time. Your breasts will be heavy with the milk you're producing for baby, and you will ache without the support of a bra. Pack at least three washable bras (five for a Caesarean); they'll need frequent washing because of your milk flow. Be sure the bras fit snugly, but get the kind with adjustable straps, since your breasts will enlarge between purchase (pre-natal) and use (post-delivery). Again, you can use up your pregnancy supply now—because within six months you'll have shrunk down to your old bra size. Naturally, if you're going to breast-feed, bring nursing bras.

Sanitary belt and pads; nursing pads. You'll need these, but many hospitals supply them. Find out.

Natural childbirth kit.

WHAT NOT TO BRING

Valuables. A surprising number of young mothers get a real obsession about being glamour girls as they glide into labor. They show up at the hospital in their best sable and every diamond they can muster.

Well, girls, forget it. That matter-of-fact nurse at the admitting desk is the only one who's going to see your baubles. She's going to take them all away from you, along with your handbag, and hide them in a nice safe locker until you're in your own bed with the baby arrived. And then you keep valuables in your room at your own risk.

It's not that hospitals are hotbeds of thievery—they're not. But every once in a while some sticky-fingered individual does make his way through the sacred halls of healing. And hospitals have enough to do, taking care of you and baby, without also keeping an eye on furs and gems and three-hundred-dollar wigs.

If you feel naked without your hairpiece or your emerald tiara—please!, the hospitals beg, try to get through labor without them. If you must have them, have your husband bring them to you the next day.

The stopwatch in your natural childbirth kit (page 104) is the only timepiece that's A-okay for the labor room. A wristwatch will go right into your safekeeping locker. So will your wedding ring, if the admitting nurse can coax it off your finger. As you may well know, among all the other swelling parts of pregnant you, count also your fingers. So if your ring has grown too tight to remove, it'll be adhesive-taped to your finger to prevent it from slipping off or getting lost in the labor and delivery rooms.

Important papers. Do not bring bankbooks, charge plates, credit cards or other such invaluable papers that are useless to you in the hospital; good only for causing worry as to their safekeeping.

Your going-home costume. Don't add these things to your hospital suitcase. For one thing, you'll just make it heavier and unwieldly—why trudge in for labor and delivery burdened down with clothes you won't need for days? Consider, also, how the weather may be totally different the morning you leave the hospital.

Your suitcase should contain only those things you'll want the moment you wake up after delivery. Anything you'll need later in your stay can be brought by your husband.

Your handbag. If you bring your handbag stuffed with money and valuable papers, someone in the admitting office will politely take it away from you. Don't try to get around it by slipping some money into a pocket instead—that too will be taken from you. Anyway, what would you do with it—tip the obstetrician? After delivery your husband can bring you the money you will need for the remainder of your hospital stay.

WHAT TO WEAR

. . . TO THE HOSPITAL

The very clothes you wear into the hospital will be stowed away in a locker until after delivery. So you might as well wear something that won't suffer from crushing, something you won't mind messing, that's comfortable to get into (probably in a hurry) and out of (ditto), and easy for your husband to take home for you after delivery (that is, not clothing that he will have to stop and fold neatly). In other words . . . your real supermarket-in-the-rain outfit. Certainly not your gala going-home costume.

And talk about taking things away from you. . . . If you remember my Introduction, I planned to enter the hospital perfectly coiffed and exquisitely manicured. Well, seems how the nurses will remove every bit of nail polish from your fingers and even your toes—because the obstetrical team will watch the color of your nail beds and toes as one of the most easily observed clues to whether you're getting enough oxygen. So forget the polish during your manicures when you're getting near due date. Painting your nails is a very easy, relaxing, pleasant pastime for the day after delivery.

Similarly, don't waste your time on a big make-up job when you're dressing for labor. The labor-room nurse will only tissue it all away and peel off your fake eyelashes. To see your physical condition properly throughout labor and delivery, the obstetrical team will want to see *you*—not your face-blusher. You can color yourself gorgeous again *after* delivery.

. . . FROM THE HOSPITAL

Leaving the hospital with her new child is one of the truly gala occasions in a woman's life, and usually she enjoys dressing for it. From about the time you pack your suitcase, start preparing your going-home costume, changing it if necessary as the weather changes. If you're in an uncertain weather period, you might want to put together two alternate costumes. Pick outfits you love, but not your skinniest pre-pregnancy clothes—some women deflate gradually.

Hang and arrange everything close together— dress or suit, coat, hat, gloves, shoes, handbag, stockings . . . everything. Show your husband where everything is (and, to be doubly sure, make a note to him), and close by place old dress- or blanket-boxes into which he can pack everything to bring to you. Then you can leave the boxes behind at the hospital, instead of having to tote home an empty suitcase along with your hospital suitcase, flowers, gifts . . . not to speak of the baby.

BABY'S GOING-HOME COSTUME

You might as well set this up at the same time as yours. If you already have the layette at home, take from it the things you'll need, and arrange them all together in a convenient place in the nursery or your bedroom.

If the layette won't arrive until after baby comes, check off the items you'll want from the following list so your husband knows what to bring.

Either way, baby's clothes can go into the same sort of cardboard box as your costume or even into a strong, clean paper shopping bag—the tiny things don't add up to a very bulky load. You will need:

1 undershirt. Short-sleeved for summer, long sleeved for winter.

2 diapers and diaper pins. In case you need to change on the way home.

1 pair rubber pants.

Socks for summer or booties for winter.

Gown or Kimono or Diaper Set or Newborn Suit or Dress.

Sweater and hat.

2 receiving blankets.

Bunting for winter.

Crib blanket for winter or crib or carriage shawl for summer.

TRANSPORTATION TO THE HOSPITAL

This is also the time to re-check instructions for getting to the hospital. Are they still valid? No blocked-off traffic routes or anything like that?

What transportation will you use? In the space below, note where your car is parked if you'll be driving; or the phone number of a relative or friend who's offered to drive you; or the phone number to call for a taxi; or the directions for a reliable, direct means of public transportation.

Find out, in the event that you'll be arriving at the hospital in the middle of the night, if any of the entrances are locked at night. Which entrance should you use? Note the location below.

....

....

....

....

....

....

....

....

....

getting your house in order

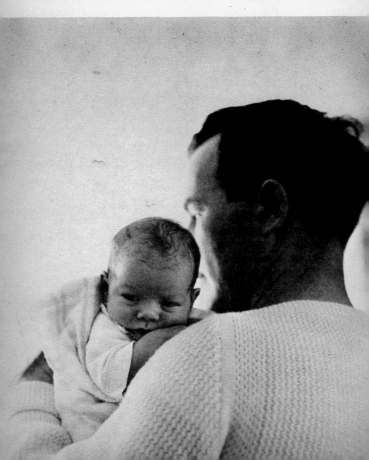

Your suitcase is packed, your hospital arrangements all made—you're ready! But what about the other members of your family? You'll be away from home for several days and you must provide ahead for all those creatures who depend on you. First of all:

OLDER CHILDREN

Arrange now for a relative, friend or housekeeper to come and care for them. Or line up people your children can stay with, preferably (for their emotional well-being) all in the same place. It's not too useful to do this too far ahead. Life is uncertain, and the best-willed promise of future availability may have to be broken because of changed circumstances. You can start lining up your stand-in early, but double-check her availability near the end of your pregnancy.

HUSBAND

Just make sure that, from now on, he always has a sufficient supply of clean laundry to see him through your absence. And if he's going to be home alone, stock the larder now with the kinds of foods he's able to manage. If he enjoys cooking, put an assortment of his favorite meats, seafoods and frozen vegetables into the freezer. If not, pre-cook a few casseroles for the freezer or buy TV dinners and the like. Add some freezable desserts and his favorite beverages. Fill the fruit section of your refrigerator. Stock up on canned soups and other hot foods he likes.

He'll be pretty rushed while you're in the hospital—visiting you and doing his own new-baby chores while still working a full schedule. Don't leave him with basic grocery shopping to do as well. If you want to be really provident, you might at the same time stock up for your first busy days back home.

Consult with your husband as you make out your shopping lists.

PLANTS & PETS

Most plants can be left safely during your hospital stay. You will have to arrange, however, for those that need frequent watering. Either take your husband or a dependable friend or relative on an instructional tour through your greenery, or board out the plants that need it. To help your substitute gardener, tape an identifying piece of colored yarn or paper to each plant pot. On a sheet of paper write down the name of each plant, its location in your house, the color of yarn taped to it, how much water each gets, how often it should be watered, and any other comments necessary.

As for pets, if necessary, arrange for boarding them. If you have someone at home who can take care of them, write out any instructions. Remember to check on your supply of pet food.

part four

post-labor labors

chapter eight

chores to complete from your hospital bed

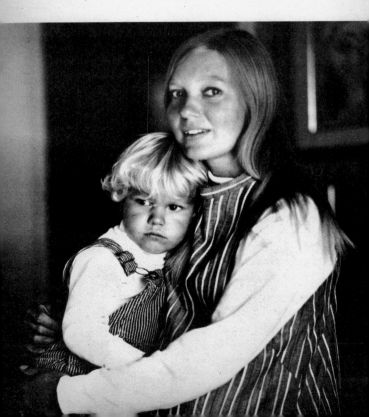

You've done it! You produced the baby. Now bask in happiness and pride, get a good rest, eat a hearty meal, do your nails, get another lovely rest, say hello to your baby, exchange congratulations with your husband, get another delicious rest. . . .

NOW! You've got four days or so to polish off last-minute chores:

Phone the painter if you've waited until now to have the baby's room painted. Your arrangements should be detailed on page 85.

Phone the birth-announcement printer if necessary. His phone number is on page 85.

Start addressing birth-announcement envelopes, checking names off the list on page 95.

Phone the people asterisked on the birth-announcement list.

Phone the godparents (see page 117).

Phone your newborn nurse if you've hired one or, if you want one and haven't yet hired one, phone an agency. Their numbers are on page 84.

Phone your domestic helpers (see page 27).

Phone those people involved in the religious ceremonies (see page 116).

Phone all the necessary numbers on your nursery planning list on page 89.

Call the diaper service listed on page 84.

Look ahead to Baby's Drugstore Shelf and Baby's Grocery Shelf and make any necessary phone calls.

BUT—do all of these things at a relaxed pace, only when and if you feel like being active. The most important thing for you now is to get as much rest as you want and your doctor advises.

If you've kept clearly detailed lists, you can easily hand all the above chores over to your husband, or parents, or in-laws, or even a kind sister or friend.

CHORES FOR THE NEW FATHER

While *you're* having the baby, *he* can make an appointment for you with the hospital hairdresser. They generally work nine-to-five on a first come, first

served basis, and are so heavily booked that unless
you act that fast you may get an appointment for
three weeks after you leave the hospital. Which could
be a tiny calamity for you if you're the kind of lady
who thinks a lady always meets her audience—and
that includes her new baby—well groomed. But have
your husband check these facts with the hospital
office first.

After the baby is born, your husband should call
your lawyer and/or accountant, if necessary, about
changing your wills or insurance, transferring stock,
setting up a trust fund, and attending to any other
legal/financial matters affecting the baby.

On the day after delivery he should come prepared—probably with a small suitcase—to take home
the clothes you wore into the hospital. At the same
time, he can bring you all the valuables you were
warned against wearing into the hospital or packing
in your suitcase. You should still keep costly items
down to a minimum, but if you're willing to take
the risk and responsibility, you can ask your husband
to bring:

A wristwatch or small clock.

Jewelry, but do try to get along with your inexpensive
costume pieces.

A handbag, a roll of dimes, and some additional
money—five or ten dollars at a time should be
enough—for phone calls, for the hairdresser, for
things like coughdrops, bobby pins, an extra nursing
bra from the hospital shop if there is one. . . .

A wig or hairpiece.

Electric curlers if the hopsital says their wiring permits it.

A portable TV, also dependent on the hospital's wiring. Get their okay first—many hospitals simply don't have sufficient electrical current in the rooms. You can always rent a set from the hospital if you'd rather not risk or bother with bringing in your own.

A small transistor radio.

Extra books, magazines, newspapers, needlework, knitting, etc.

As you can see, your husband will have his hands full too. So try to keep all the information he'll need in one place. Check off those items you'll want him to bring and enter them on his list—when the time comes, you can tear it out and give it to him. Fill in all that you can before you go to the hospital, and the rest you can do at your bedside.

CHORES FOR THE NEW FATHER

....

....

....

....

....

Calls to make

....

....

....

....

....

....

Errands to run

....

....

....

....

Shopping list

....

....

....

....

....

....

....

Things to bring to the hospital

....

....

....

....

....

Notes on where to find what

....

....

....

....

....

PHOTOGRAPHING YOUR NEWBORN

This is the chore—no, pleasure, of course!—most new fathers think of first. But generally they're persuaded to let the hospital provide baby's very earliest camera studies. Your hospital may ask you, long before you enter, to pre-order first-day photos of your baby. But even if you don't do so, they'll likely take some pictures anyway, and ask you afterward if you want prints.

The hospital prefers using its own photographer for several reasons. First of all, he has a special machine that takes excellent pictures without using a flash which would be damaging to a newborn's eyes. Then, too, the nurses can gauge the best, least disturbing time for baby to make his camera debut. Usually this is on his second day—occasionally on the first—and the developed shots are shown to you and your husband no later than the following day for your approval. The finished prints are ready by the time you leave the hospital, or sent to your home shortly thereafter. (Premature babies are not photographed until they attain a five-pound weight.)

If your husband would like to take his own photos of the baby even so, he should certainly plan on not using a flash, and he should get exact instructions from the nursery personnel.

By the way, if you don't already have a good still camera and movie camera, as proud parents you'll want them now. Think about adding them to your Rich Uncle list on page 99. You might even think about adding a tape-recorder, so you can compile a complete audio-visual scrapbook.

BABY'S DRUGSTORE SHELF

Whoever is going to be helping you with baby at

home—a nurse, a relative, a neighbor, or Daddy— get that person to shop for the following baby-care items during the days before you get home:

Mild soap or baby cleanser
Baby shampoo
* Baby oil
Baby powder
Baby lotion

Sterile cotton
Cotton balls
* Cotton swabs
Baby brush and comb (may come as a gift)

The hospital nurses or your pediatrician may suggest additions.

BABY'S GROCERY SHELF

That would be you—wouldn't it?—if you're breast-feeding. If not, you'll need a number of bottle-feeding accessories. Buy these ahead if you're sure you'll be bottle-feeding; or have someone do it before you arrive home if you've waited to decide.

8 to 10 8-ounce bottles for milk
2 to 4 4-ounce bottles for juice or water
bottle brush, nipple brush
extra nipples
bottle sterilizer
bottle warmer

tongs
bottle caps and covers
can opener
funnel
32-ounce pitcher

The following items may come in as gifts by the

---

* Some doctors have reservations about these two products. Check with your pediatrician.

time baby is ready for them. If they don't, you can always pick them up at a neighborhood variety store on short notice when you need them:

Feeding dish
Feeding spoons
Bibs
Training cup

As for materials for baby's milk formula. . . . The hospital nursery will make you a farewell gift of a 24-hour supply of formula for baby's first day home. Plus instructions for carrying on yourself. Take notes here.

----

chapter nine

going home

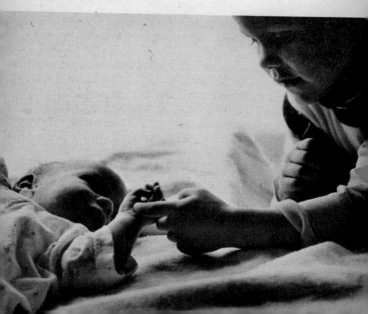

HOSPITAL FAREWELL

Almost always this is between baby's ten A.M. and two P.M. feedings. For the homeward journey, the nursery will give you formula for bottle-fed babies or a bottle or two of glucose water if you're breast-feeding.

Your preparations for leaving start the day before, with your husband taking on a whole new array of chores for the occasion. When he comes for his last evening visit, he brings baby's going-home costume so you can check the box to see if everything's there, and so it's sure to be ready in your room early the next morning when a nurse comes to get the clothes for dressing baby.

Your husband should also bring your going-home costume. Listen to weather forecasts during the day, and phone to tell him which outfit you will want. But if an expensive fur coat is part of your costume, you can certainly wait for that until he arrives next morning to escort you out the door.

On that last evening he should take home some of the heavier things you can do without now: books, needlework, electric curlers. . . . Perhaps also the gifts that may have arrived at the hospital. And flowers that may still be fresh enough to dress up your first days back home—though you might instead like to send your extra flowers to the children's ward or to elderly chronic patients.

Your husband will also arrange transportation for getting you all home. And if, despite all your planning, on the morning you leave you still have to take some gifts and flowers along with you—he should take that into account in his transportation arrangements.

If someone else will be joining your going-home group, phone them the day before to get everything set. A newborn nurse, for instance, usually moves into your home at least a day before you return there, to settle herself in before she has to concentrate on the baby. So probably she'll join your husband on his way to the hospital that last morning.

DO YOU TIP THE NURSES?

Nurses don't expect it, and may very well refuse money if you offer it. If one or two nurses have been particularly helpful, it would be more gracious to express your gratitude with a small personal gift instead—a pretty handkerchief, a tiny flask of perfume, a good-looking coin purse. . . . Most appreciated of all: a letter to the supervisor, commending the nurses you especially liked. Your words will adorn their career records for eternity.

THE POST-PARTUM BLUES

After you get home, and the first fine flush of motherhood subsides, if you're like two-thirds of all new mothers you're going to be depressed. Some of you only for a few days, some of you on and off for months. Some will start feeling depressed while still in the hospital. Some of you will find yourselves going on long crying jags, others will just feel a little forlorn sometimes. But all of you, except for one woman in a thousand, will snap out of it naturally by the time baby is several months old—and that one woman will be fine after a few talks with an understanding psychiatrist.

The reasons for the blues are many. 1) Your body, after all, has just undergone a pretty overwhelming series of hormone changes which affect your personality. 2) You're suddenly working quite hard, taking care of a demanding new baby . . . you're tired. 3) You're worried about whether you're doing everything right for the baby. 4) Emotionally, there's a letdown after the tremendous anticipation in pregnancy—and, psychologists say, the new mother unconsciously feels a temporary sense of loss when the baby leaves her body to start its independent life. In fact, recent studies show that most women do not feel an immediate surge of love when they first see their babies. It takes a while.

Wow! If you weren't depressed before, you are now—now that you know how many good reasons you have. But it'll all go away, for an equal number of good reasons:

1) Your hormone balance will return—keep visiting your obstetrician until he discharges you.

2) You're going to get as much rest and sleep as you can. And if you've used this book correctly, you've prepared so well for motherhood that you're not exhausting yourself with extra chores in the post-partum period.

3) You took the parenthood class, I hope, so you do know how to take care of your baby. (Studies show that women who attend such classes with their husbands are far less likely to suffer the post-partum blues than women who attend alone or not at all.)

4) You're going to be perfectly delighted with the baby outside your body, as he begins to respond and react and think and do and learn . . . to be your child instead of your Bump. Most new mothers really fall in love with their babies when they're between six and nine weeks old. Generally it's that first smile that does it.

And a few things extra: You'll be resuming your sex life, at your doctor's signal. You will remember the Beauty chapter, and keep yourself looking pretty for your continued but not too hectic social life. You'll do sit-ups and whatever else your obstetrician recommends to get back a morale-lifting figure.

And you'll put this book away and move on to the capable hands of your pediatrician and your baby-care manual. And your baby-sitters:

BABY-SITTERS LIST

NAME	PHONE NUMBER	COMMENTS

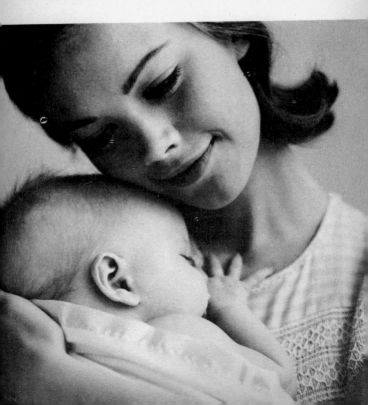

chapter ten

memories to look back on

Your pregnancy will always be remembered, but nothing brings back memories as well—evokes the time and the place and how you were feeling then and there—as your own personal diary. Why not record events that were meaningful to you. The day you found out you were definitely pregnant. The place where you ate dinner to celebrate. The first thing your husband said when you told him—and how *you* were feeling about it too. The first time the baby kicked. And maybe a few words about how you felt month to month—not just physically, but emotionally. Write down what it was like when you saw your baby for the very first time. Do use the next few pages. Date your entries; they needn't be long, a sentence or two will bring it all back.

1 pair rubber pants

Socks for summer or booties for winter